A WOMAN'S DISEASE

A WOMAN'S DISEASE

The History of Cervical Cancer

Ilana Löwy

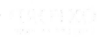

OXFORD

A WOMAN'S DISEASE

The History of Cervical Cancer

⚬⚬⚬

Ilana Löwy

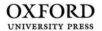

OXFORD
UNIVERSITY PRESS

OXFORD
UNIVERSITY PRESS

Great Clarendon Street, Oxford OX2 6DP

Oxford University Press is a department of the University of Oxford.
It furthers the University's objective of excellence in research, scholarship,
and education by publishing worldwide in

Oxford New York

Auckland Cape Town Dar es Salaam Hong Kong Karachi
Kuala Lumpur Madrid Melbourne Mexico City Nairobi
New Delhi Shanghai Taipei Toronto

With offices in

Argentina Austria Brazil Chile Czech Republic France Greece
Guatemala Hungary Italy Japan Poland Portugal Singapore
South Korea Switzerland Thailand Turkey Ukraine Vietnam

Oxford is a registered trade mark of Oxford University Press
in the UK and in certain other countries

Published in the United States
by Oxford University Press Inc., New York

© Ilana Löwy 2011

British Library Cataloguing in Publication Data

Data available

Library of Congress Cataloging in Publication Data

Data available

Typeset by SPI Publisher Services, Pondicherry, India
Printed in Great Britain
on acid-free paper by
Clays Ltd, St Ives plc

ISBN 978-0-19-954881-1

1 3 5 7 9 10 8 6 4 2

CONTENTS

ACKNOWLEDGEMENTS

I'm very grateful to Helen and Bill Bynum for persuading me to write this book, "forcing" me to venture into unknown territories and to learn many new things, and providing unfailing encouragement and support. I am as always thankful to my home institution, INSERM, the French Institute of Health and Medical Research, which has afforded continual support for my atypical investigations, and to my research center, CERMES 3, which provides excellent intellectual and material conditions for my work, as well as rich possibilities for confronting my ideas with those of other scholars studying intersections between science, medicine and society.

This study benefited greatly from exchanges with many colleagues, from the rapidly growing though unofficial history of cancer network. Thanks to all the participants in the conferences on cancer history in Washington, Manchester, and Paris, and to scholars who made these conferences possible: Isabelle Baszanger David Cantor, John Pickstone and Carsten Timmermann. Special thanks to Robert Aronowitz, Yolanda Eraso, Ornella Mosccuci and Elisabeth Toon, who generously shared with me their knowledge of the history of cervical cancer.

In Brazil, Luiz Antonio Teixeira helped me to understand the specificity of efforts to prevent cervical cancer in that country, and Claudia Bonan, Marilena Correa, Andrea Loyola and Katia da Silva taught me about problems of women's reproductive health in a developing country.

Some of the material in this book draws on my own original research published in an earlier book *Preventive Strikes* (Johns Hopkins University Press, 2009) and the following articles:

- Ilana Löwy, 'Cancer, women and public health: the history of screening for cervical cancer', *Manguinhos*, 2010, 17 (supl. 1): 53-67.
- Luiz Antonio Teixiera and Ilana Löwy, 'Imperfect tools for a difficult job: Colposcopy, 'colpocytology' and screening for cervical cancer in Brazil', *Social Studies of Medicine*, in press.
- Ilana Löwy, '"Because of Their Praiseworthy Modesty, They Consult Too Late": Regime of Hope and Cancer of the Womb, 1800–1910', *Bulletin of the History of Medicine*, 2011, 85-356-383.

I'm grateful to Latha Menon at the Oxford University Press for her support for this project, to Emma Marchant for her highly efficient help in bringing this volume to press, to Nick Prowse for careful copy editing of the manuscript, and to Fiona Vlemmiks for dealing with the final stage of production.

Thanks to my extended family for being there for me when needed, a permanent intellectual stimulation , and for putting my (hopefully mild) obsessions into perspective.

During the writing of this book I prematurely lost two close colleagues and friends: Olga Amsterdamska, who died in August, 2009, and Harry Marks, who died in January, 2011. Their high intellectual standards, sharp but always positive criticism, and their unfailing support, sustained my scholarship. In the last stages of the production of this book I repeatedly found myself thinking that I should ask Olga and/or Harry to help me to clarify this or that point—then realized with a pang the extent of the loss, for me and for our scholarly communities.

PROLOGUE:
THREE PATIENTS

Three well-known women—Byron's daughter and computing pioneer Ada Lovelace (1815–1852), the Argentinian performer, politician, and First Lady Eva Péron (1919–1952), and the television personality Jade Goody (1981–2009)—died young from a painful and devastating disease: cancer of the uterus. Two of them, Eva Péron and Jade Goody, suffered from the most frequent form of this malignancy, cancer of the uterine cervix. Descriptions of Ada Lovelace's disease indicate that she might have suffered from the same disease, but in the mid nineteenth century the distinct entity 'cervical cancer' did not yet exist. Comparison of stories of these three women makes visible radical changes in the understanding, prevention, and treatment of cervical cancer in 150 years. It also points to important continuities in the history of this disease.

Ada Lovelace

Augusta Ada Byron, the Countess of Lovelace, was born in 1815, from Byron's short marriage to Anna Isabella (Anabella) Milbank. Her parents separated when she was a baby, and she never met her father, who died when she was 9 years old. Her mother provided her with a mathematic and scientific education, an attempt to neutralize the hereditary influence of Byron's 'madness'. Married at the age of 20 to Lord Lovelace (William King, 1805–1893), she quickly produced two sons and a daughter. Marriage and maternity did not dampen her interest in mathematics. Through one of her teachers, Mary Somerville, she met the mathematician and pioneer of computing, Charles Babbage (1791–1871). The two became friends and part-time collaborators. Lovelace's detailed notes to her translation of a memoir on Babbage's 'analytical machine', written by the Italian mathematician Luigi Manebrea, led to her posthumous reputation as a pioneer of computer programming. Not all the historians of computing agree with this view. For some, Babbage and Lovelace did not play a significant role in the development of computers, and Ada Lovelace's famous notes were closer to a poetic vision than to a blueprint for a working device. On the other hand, these notes seem to grasp the hidden potential of mechanic calculation; this alone may legitimate her—and Babbage's—posthumous fame.

Ada Lovelace suffered from poor health. In her teens she was paralysed for a year following a measles attack, and all her life she was plagued by severe headaches, poor vision, digestive troubles, and a 'weak heart'. A life of sickness was an acceptable style of Victorian femininity, but Lovelace went further and claimed that her ailments and her mathematical powers were intimately connected. Her bodily complaints, she explained, provided her with a 'laboratory' to explore the corporeal conditions for producing knowledge and allowed her to develop a 'calculus of the nervous system'. In the Victorian period, women's bodies were seen as too weak for a powerful mental effort. Men from Lovelace's entourage were worried that her mathematical studies were destroying her health. Lovelace turned this proposal on its head. She attempted to transform her multiple ailments into raw material for her studies, and produced copious notes on mind–body connections.

Until 1851 Ada Lovelace suffered from multiple, poorly defined symptoms, attributed to her weak constitution. In spring 1851, she developed a precise ailment: a violent haemorrhage. One of the physicians who examined Ada, Dr Lee, strongly suspected a uterine malignancy and conveyed his fears to her husband, Lord Lovelace. However, her other doctors proposed different and less threatening explanations, such as an intermittent fever. Ada Lovelace's personal physician, Dr John Locock, and another consultant, Dr Malcolm, prescribed quinine, nitrate of silver, rest, and avoidance of writing. Locock also prescribed leeching for the 'local depletion' of the sore that produced the bleeding, and consumption of wine and other restoratives to make up for her loss of blood. Lovelace's mother attributed her disease to overexcitement. Ada Lovelace herself blamed 'miserable East Winds', high pressure of life of the times, and the general state of society.

Ada Lovelace faithfully followed Dr Locock's prescriptions, but her health continued to deteriorate. She had frequent haemorrhages, developed chronic pain, and was obliged to use an 'invalid chair', with wheels of India rubber, to move around. Dr Locock performed in July 1851 an internal examination, which at that was time an unusual step to be undertaken only in very severe cases. He had found 'an extensive and deep-seated sore' in her genital organs (a clinical description which may indicate that Ada Lovelace suffered from a cervical tumour, accessible by physical examination). Nevertheless, Locock reassured Lovelace that she had a 'healthy sore' (that is, one that could be cured) and maintained his previous treatment. He also prescribed her camphor pills to control convulsions, and opium to alleviate her pain. Ada Lovelace's mother objected to the use of narcotics, and proposed a mesmerist cure. The latter was not very successful; Lovelace wrote to her mother in early 1852 that she had gone back to her 'old friend' opium, because mesmerism seemed to be powerless when she suffered from a violent pain. She also experimented with cannabis, and reluctantly agreed to be treated with chloroform when her pain became too strong.[1]

In spite of her rapidly worsening condition, Ada Lovelace remained optimistic. In winter 1851–1852 she continued her correspondence with Babbage, and hoped to resume her scientific work. In the spring, however, her pain intensified and she became increasingly weak. In July 1852 a new symptom appeared, a hard swelling of the uterus. Dr Locock was very worried by it, and sent for a new consultant, Dr West, who examined Ada Lovelace on 28 July. West announced to Lord Lovelace that Dr Lee's initial diagnosis was correct: Ada was suffering from a fatal disease, and her days were numbered. Lord Lovelace immediately transmitted this message to his wife, asking her to leave all her affairs in order.[2] Even before West's announcement, Ada Lovelace herself realized that she was going to die. She had written her will, started to talk about her funeral, and expressed a wish to see her sons, Ralph and Byron, who at that time no longer lived with her.

In her final months Ada Lovelace suffered attacks of agony and delirium. Maddened by pain that could no longer be controlled entirely by opiates, she could not be held in bed and threw herself against the furniture or on the floor. The room was then padded with mattresses to prevent her causing future injury to herself. When the pain relented, she would fall into a fretful sleep on the floor; then the pain would resume and she would writhe around in agony. She decided at this point to stay on the floor. She was later removed to a fracture bed, parts of which could be tilted to increase the patient's comfort. Her family, including her younger son Byron, witnessed her extreme suffering; Byron stayed in her room and sponged her face with water during the ever-shorter respites from pain.

On 29 August Ada had a seizure and convulsions and doctors believed she had only a few hours to live. But on the next day she revived. She continued to hover between convulsions, delirium, semi-conscious state, and lucidity. Dr West wrote a detailed account of Lovelace's case in which he bluntly stated that the cancer had invaded the internal organs, causing untreatable anguish. In November her agony increased and her symptoms included vomiting; her mother wrote that her intestines had been invaded by the disease, and that the pain extended through her whole alimentary canal, describing the situation as 'horrible'. Ada Lovelace's attendant, Miss Fitzhugh, described her agony as alternation between fainting and fierce pains. On the night of 27–28 November 1852 Ada Lovelace entered a coma after long fit of convulsions and died without regaining consciousness. Dr West reported that her last moments were peaceful. Ada Lovelace's obituary in *The Times* praised the patience and fortitude with which she had borne her last illness. It did not mention her contributions to the construction of calculating machines or other intellectual endeavours.

Eva Péron

Eva Maria Ibarguren Duarte was born in 1919, probably in the Argentinian town of Los Toldos. An illegitimate child of a mother of modest origins, she became in the early 1940s a popular actress and radio personality. In 1945 she married the Argentinian politician Juan Péron (1895–1974). In 1946 Juan Péron was elected president of the Argentinian republic. Eva Péron (Evita, 'the little Eve', to her followers and admirers) became one of the leaders of the Peronist movement, and skilfully used the radio to advance the movement's cause. Eva Péron promoted women's right to vote, was deeply involved in charity work, and became a passionate defender of the interests of the poor (the *decamisados*, or 'shirtless' people). She also became, especially after her premature death, a Peronist icon and a 'secular saint'. Peronism divides and continues to divide the Argentinians, and narratives of Eva Péron's disease and death are often strongly coloured by the author's political opinions. There are several conflicting stories about her cancer, and some details remain unclear. The general outline of the history of her illness is, however, well documented.

In January 1949 Eva Péron, who suffered from abdominal pains, underwent an operation for appendicitis, performed by Dr Oscar Ivanissevich. Ivanissevich did not find an inflammation of the appendix. He later claimed that he suspected uterine disease, but Eva Péron refused further investigations, fearing a conspiracy to sabotage her political ascension.[3] This story has an interesting twist. Many years earlier, Eva Péron's mother was diagnosed with a uterine tumour, and was successfully operated on by Ivanissevich; she survived her daughter.

In 1950 and 1951, Eva Péron was frantically occupied with various political actions and was deeply involved in the management of her foundation, destined to help the poor. She was also expected to become vice president of Argentina, a move blocked later by the oligarchy and the military. According to her collaborators, Eva Péron believed at that time that she did not have time to be sick, and elected to ignore bleeding, fainting spells, and pain.

In September 1951 Eva Péron's health deteriorated to the point that she could not deny her problems any more and agreed to undergo a gynaecological examination under general anaesthesia. This examination, made on 26 September by the gynaecologist Humberto Dionisi, revealed an extended cancer of the cervix. The diagnosis was confirmed by biopsy (analysis of a slice of tissue fixed, stained, and observed under a microscope) made by the pathologist Lascano Gonzalez. Eva Péron's doctors, Humberto Dionisi and Jeorge Albertelli, proposed an aggressive treatment: first radiation therapy with radium-containing needles and blood transfusions to make Péron stronger, then, as soon as possible, a radical hysterectomy (ablation of the womb and surrounding tissues).

Juan Péron, informed about his wife's diagnosis, was devastated by the news, probably even more so because his first wife, Aurelia Tizon, had died at the age of 28 from a cervical malignancy. (Today cervical cancer is linked with a viral infection; it is possible that Eva Péron was infected by her husband with a cancer-inducing virus.) He decided to ask the opinion of a known US specialist, Dr George Pack. Pack was brought secretly to Buenos Aires, and on 26 October met Eva Péron's doctor, Albertelli, and two additional Argentinian specialists, Dr Mendé and Dr Abel Canonico. A document signed by the four doctors explicitly stated that Eva Péron's prognosis was 'reserved', because the patient had had symptoms for a long time, and due to her young age, the size of the lesions, their histological nature, and the strong suspicion of invasion of the tissues around the uterus by malignant cells.[4] The consulted doctors also agreed that hysterectomy should not be delayed any more, in spite of Eva Péron's persisting weakness.

Eva Péron underwent surgical ablation of the uterus on 6 November 1951. George Pack, who returned to the USA after the consultation, was brought back to operate on Péron. She was not aware of this fact: officially her surgeon was Dr Ricardo Fionchettino. Pack saw her only when under anaesthesia, and left the operating theatre after ending his task. George Pack's involvement in Péron's treatment was well known by the US embassy and the CIA, which had a direct interest in the potential effects of Eva Péron's disease on Argentinian politics. The news was also leaked to the US press: *Newsweek* speculated about Pack's possible role in treating an important 'foreign politician'.[5] Eva Péron's surgery confirmed a reserved prognosis. The cancer was present in tissues in the vicinity of the womb and Eva Péron's surgeons were not sure whether they had been able to take out all of the cancerous tissue. Worse, analysis of the excised material by the pathologist Grato Bur showed the presence of a metastasis near the ovary. This finding indicated that Eva's case was hopeless: there was no cure for cervical cancer that had spread to distant organs (and this is still true).[6]

Eva Péron was not told what her disease was, although she might have suspected the truth. She recovered from the surgery and radiation therapy and in January 1952 resumed her political activity. However, the respite was short. Pain and bleeding returned in February. During spring and summer 1952 Eva Péron stayed most of the day in her bed, although she made a few political speeches, which became increasingly more violent and desperate.

At that time her disease became public knowledge, and her followers sent her flowers, amulets, and miraculous images. Péron's doctors tried to stop the cancer's progress with additional radiation therapy. They also attempted chemotherapy with nitrogen mustard, at that time an innovative therapeutic approach. These efforts were unsuccessful. By June 1952 Eva Péron weighed only 38 kg, and her faithful assistant, Atilla Renzi, unscrewed the regulating wheel of her scales to hide her weight loss. There were persistent rumours in the presidential palace that Juan Péron could not stand the odours emanating from his wife's dying body. Some of his aids reported that he entered her room very rarely, and when he did he kept a muslin mask over his face, like a bee keeper.[7]

Eva Péron was treated with high doses of narcotics to control her pain, and in May and June 1952 was only intermittently lucid. Nevertheless, on 1 May she dragged herself to the balcony of the presidential palace to make her last political speech, and on 4 June, when Juan Péron started his second presidential term, she accompanied her husband during his trip by car from their residence to the Congress. She was given a triple dose of morphine and was able to stand in the open presidential car thanks to a plaster support and a belt, both hidden by her fur coat.

Eva pretended to believe people who told her she would get well soon. Juan Péron even asked his wife's tailor to visit her one week before her death, to show her samples of tissue to prepare clothes for a forthcoming trip to Europe. In fact, she was probably fully aware that she was dying. She took leave from her friends, distributed her jewellery and other personal effects among them, and mentioned her nearing demise to people close to her. In her last weeks Eva Péron prepared a collection of her speeches, *My Message*, meant to be her political testament, and wrote two different versions of her will, one official, passing everything to Juan Péron and the Argentinian people, and another, much more personal and desperate. The second will was never published.

On 18 July Eva Péron went into a coma, and was generally believed to be dying. She woke up, however, and even walked a few steps on Juan's arm. After this experience, her doctors did not hide the truth about her disease any more, and discovered that she was knowledgeable about cervical cancer. On 25 July two German specialists, Paul Uhlenbruck from Cologne and Heinrich Kalk from Kassel, were flown from Germany for a last-ditch consultation. They had told Juan Péron that nothing more could be done for his wife. She died the following day, on 26 July. Eva Péron's funeral was accompanied by dramatic manifestations of popular grief. Crowds totally blocked the streets of Buenos Aires during her funeral. Six people were trampled to death and nearly 2000 were injured in the rush to see Eva Péron's body.

Jade Goody

The British television personality Jade Cerisa Lorraine Goody was born in 1981 in Bermondsey, South London. The only child of two drug addicts (her father died from a drug overdose) she had a chaotic childhood and limited education. Goody, who trained to be a dental assistant, became known to the UK public through the third series of the television programme *Big Brother*. Her outspokenness and candour won her public favour and notoriety, although she was also criticized by the media for her ignorance and occasionally improper behaviour. In an especially damaging episode, she addressed racial slurs to an Indian actress who participated with her in the programme *Celebrity*

Big Brother in 2007. The controversy over this and other similar episodes did not put an end to Jade Goody's media career. She appeared frequently in articles in gossip-oriented magazines, at one point had her own reality television show and magazine column, opened a beauty salon, and successfully launched a fragrance.[8]

In August 2008, when Jade Goody was participating in an Indian version of *Big Brother* named *Big Boss* (part of an effort to erase the negative impact of her racist remarks), she collapsed several times during the show and was diagnosed with cervical cancer. She had previously been told about her abnormal Pap smears (a test that detects precancerous lesions of the cervix; see Chapter 4 in this volume), but had failed to act on this information. When Jade returned to the UK in early September she learned that she was suffering from advanced cancer. She underwent surgical ablation of the womb, radiotherapy, and chemotherapy. However, the treatment failed to arrest the tumour's rapid progress. In February 2009 Goody learned that her cancer had spread to her bowels and liver. Her doctors informed her that she only had a short time to live, and switched to exclusively palliative care, which included severing some of her nerves to limit cancer-induced pain. The news of her poor prognosis was publicized widely by the media, with Jade Goody's active participation. She sold rights for exclusive coverage of her treatment, her marriage to her partner, Jack Tweed, and her christening to the UK tabloid newspapers, explaining that she wished before her death to raise as much money as possible for her two young sons. Jade Goody died on 22 March 2009.

Jade Goody's disease and death attracted attention to the issue of cervical cancer and to the importance of screening for this disease. The publicity surrounding Jade's cancer persuaded many UK women to undergo a Pap smear. She was proud of this effect, and her publicist, Max Clifford, claimed that she had already saved the lives of countless young women. Jade Goody's predicament promoted a review of the UK National Health Service's rule to start screening for cervical cancer only at the age of 25. The panel that reviewed this rule decided, however, to keep the original guidelines, arguing that the screening of younger women would produce more harm than good.[9]

One of the recurring themes in debates on Jade Goody's very public disease and death was the extent of her own responsibility for her fate. Goody recognized that she had ignored previous warnings. She had received positive Pap-smear results together with urgent calls to attend hospital for treatment, but had failed to do so. The reason for her seemingly irrational behaviour, she explained in an interview after her cancer diagnosis, was fear of repeating a painful experience. She had had an abnormal Pap smear when she was 16 years old and underwent treatment to remove precancerous cells. The 'burning' of these cells 'nearly traumatized me for life, it was so painful'.[10] When she had heard again that her Pap smear had shown abnormal cells she consequently refused to be treated and ignored her doctors' warnings. Debates on Jade Goody's cancer have often focused on the importance of regular Pap smears. A few commentators noted that the problem was not that Goody did not have cervical smears—she had many such tests—but that, through her own negligence or lack of persistence by health professionals, or both, she failed to receive appropriate treatment after a positive Pap smear.

Jade Goody's death was seen by some commentators as exemplary and praiseworthy, because she was very open about her diagnosis, gradually worsening prognosis, effects of cancer treatments, and forthcoming death. Other commentators were disturbed by the fact that Jade Goody sold to the popular press the exclusive rights for her pictures in the last weeks of her life. Some journalists stressed that Jade Goody died tragically young, while others underlined that she died from a (presumably) preventable disease, and that, to an important extent, she was responsible for her own fate. Images of the severely ill Jade Goody, omnipresent in the British media in February and March 2009, were difficult to stabilize: they hovered between pity and faint contempt, the admirable and the suspicious, a display of the universality of suffering and the particularities of British tabloid culture, praise of modern medicine and bemoaning its impotence. The avalanche of media reports about Jade's terminal disease also masked an unease about the disease from which she was dying: a malignant tumour which destroys women's reproductive organs.

Continuity and change

The stories of disease of Ada Lovelace, Eva Péron, and Jade Goody are at the same time very different and quite similar. Ada Lovelace was at first diagnosed with a poorly defined disease of the womb. Her treatment, grounded in the principle of purification through bleeding and fortification through the administration of tonics, was similarly non-specific: the same remedies were prescribed for a wide range of pathologies. Only when her disease progressed was she told that she had a deadly malignant tumour of the womb. A hundred years later, Eva Péron underwent a clinical examination and a biopsy, and was diagnosed with a well-defined disease: cervical cancer. She received a specific treatment: radiation therapy, surgical removal of the womb, and rudimentary chemotherapy. Eva Péron was never explicitly told what her disease was, although in all probability she knew that she suffered from an advanced malignancy. Jade Goody was first diagnosed with a precancerous condition and later with a confirmed cervical cancer. She was immediately informed about her diagnosis and prognosis. Her treatment—surgery, radiation therapy, and chemotherapy—was not very different from Eva Péron's treatment more than half a century earlier, although Goody received more advanced forms of these cancer therapies, especially chemotherapy. The main difference, however, was elsewhere. Eva Péron's disease was presented as a random disaster. By contrast, many commentators believed that Jade Goody brought her fate on herself. Thanks to the extension of screening for cervical lesions, cervical cancer is presented in the twenty-first century as a preventable disease.

The stories of Ada Lovelace, Eva Péron, and Jade Goody show the extent and the limits of medical progress. It is possible to detect precancerous changes in the cervix, and in many cases prevent the development of a cervical malignancy. Once the cancer spreads from the womb to other tissues and organs the chances of its cure are, however, slim. Ada Lovelace, who, according to present-day criteria, received an inefficient and possibly harmful treatment, lived for a year and half after the appearance of her first typical symptoms, whereas Eva Péron and Jade Goody, treated with multiple resources of modern medicine, lived, respectively, 11 and 10 months after their diagnoses. Looking from the point of view of a woman with a disseminated cancer of the cervix, the main advance made by medicine in the last century and half is the development of more efficient ways to alleviate the distressing manifestations of this disease.

Ada Lovelace's and Eva Péron's cancer acquired meaning through its intersection with their lives. Ada Lovelace's disease was apprehended mainly through its effects on her relationships with a powerful mother and famous friends, and that of Eva Péron through its influence on Argentinian politics. This is partly true for Jade Goody's cancer too. Her highly public disease mirrored her media persona. In addition, however, stories about Jade Goody's suffering and death were interwoven with detailed descriptions of prevention and treatment of cervical tumours. People who read them learned about Jade Goody's achievements, problems, family, and friends, but also about cervical smears, screening campaigns, elimination of precancerous lesions, and treatment of advanced malignancies. In the twenty-first century, cervical cancer itself became the 'hero' of the story.

1

THE EARLY HISTORY
OF TUMOURS OF THE WOMB

On wombs and women

In the twenty-first century cervical cancer no longer occupies an important place on the list of diseases dreaded by Western women. Breast cancer is everywhere, but cervical cancer is barely visible. The death of Jade Goody produced a spike of interest in screening for cervical cancer in Britain. However, a few months later screening levels returned to those seen prior to the so-called 'Goody effect'. UK commentators had noted that Goody's disease made women aware of the fact that cervical cancer can kill. Such a remainder was not necessary a century and half ago. At that time 'cancer of the womb', a term that included cancer of the cervix and of the uterine body (today, endometrial cancer), was the first cause of women's death from malignant tumours, and a universally dreaded disease.

In the nineteenth century cancer was seen as a female ailment. The main malignancies in women, of the breast and uterus, produced typical symptoms, especially in advanced stages. This was not the case with tumours equally frequent in both sexes or those more frequent in men. People who died from cancers of internal organs—stomach, colon, lung, liver, kidney, or pancreas—were rarely diagnosed with malignant tumours. They suffered from an acute digestive failure, blood congestion, pulmonary ailments, chronic pain, increasing weakness, loss of appetite, and wasting, and sometimes simply from 'old age'. By contrast, it was difficult to miss dramatic changes in a cancer-affected breast, or the uncontrolled blood loss and vaginal secretions that appeared in advanced cancer of the womb. French mortality data from the 1830s reveal that cancer was diagnosed two and half times more often in women that in men. Approximately 80% of women reported to have died from cancer had a tumour of either the uterus or the breast, with the former malignancy approximately twice as frequent as the latter. Data collected in the mid nineteenth century by the Registrar General in England shows a similar excess of women's cancer deaths, and a similar distribution of female cancers. In England, women died mainly from cancers of the uterus and breast, with uterine cancer approximately two and a half times more frequent than breast cancer.

Death registries provide the only data on the occurrence of uterine tumours in the nineteenth century. With the generalization of microscopic diagnosis of cancer disease in the early twentieth century, a definitive diagnosis of a malignant tumour was made by pathologists who studied fixed and stained tissues under the microscope (this is still true in the twenty-first century). Without a microscopic diagnosis it is sometimes impossible to know whether a disease described as 'cancer' on the basis of its clinical signs was a malignant growth as defined today. Early stages of 'cancer of the womb' could have been easily confused with other gynaecological diseases: syphilitic lesions, other venereal diseases, ulcers, or benign tumours.

On the other hand, an advanced cancer of the uterus produced very often characteristic manifestations. Retrospective diagnosis is a perilous enterprise, especially in the absence of materials (cadavers, conserved tissues) that can be examined with modern laboratory techniques. Nevertheless, when a women died with typical symptoms of 'cancer of the womb'—and only in that case—is it reasonable to assume that she had indeed suffered from a malignant tumour.

Doctors and malignant tumours of the womb

From antiquity onwards, doctors were interested in women's reproductive organs. Women were valorized through their capacity to produce healthy children, especially male heirs, and nearly all their health problems were related to their reproductive organs, above all the uterus. The distinctive, and highly distressing symptoms of advanced uterine tumours attracted the attention of some doctors of Antiquity, the Middle Ages, the Renaissance, and the Enlightenment. An Egyptian papyrus from 1700 BC described a disease of the womb that might have been a malignant tumour. There are possible allusions to uterine tumours in Hippocratic writings (fourth century BC), and in Hindu manuscripts from approximately the same period. Greek sources mention the Greek surgeon Philoxenus of Alexandria (c.75 BC), who had a reputation as an expert on tumours, especially in women, while Latin ones describe the activities of Roman physician Soranus (AD 98–138), one of the first to mention the use of an instrument called a *dioptra*—probably akin to a speculum—employed to examine patients with abnormal vaginal bleeding and ulcers of the womb. The classical writing of Galen (AD 29–c.210) includes a description that may refer to a cancerous uterus.

The Roman doctor Oribasius (c. AD 325–403) advocated cauterization in cases of 'malignant thymus' of the womb. The author of a late Roman gynaecological study, Aetius of Amida (AD 502–575), was more conservative and advised against surgery for such 'malignant thymus' or 'polypus'. Aetius summarized available information on 'uterine chancres', and divided them into ulcerative and non-ulcerative types. His writings were copied during the Middle Ages, and were considered the main source of information on diseases of female genital organs. There were no new developments in this domain until the Renaissance, when the French doctor Ambroise Paré (1510–1590) employed a speculum (an oblong instrument inserted into the vagina) to examine an ulcerated cervix. Paré recommended the amputation of such a diseased cervix, but probably did not act upon this recommendation. He also designed a metal device which facilitated the free passage of uterine discharges. Nikolaas Tulpius (1593–1674) is credited with the first successful surgical removal of the cervix. The surgery was considered highly dangerous, and therefore was very rare. In his 1762 *Treatise on the Diseases of Women* Jean Astruc (1684–1766) described pelvic inflammatory disease and 'tumours of the cervix', which included malignant and non-malignant growths. The distinction between these two types of growth was made on the basis of the patients' ultimate fate: increasing invalidity which led to death was a proof of malignancy. This principle was already present in the writing of the Roman medical writer Celsus, who explained that 'to distinguish a benign tumour that can be cured from a cancer that cannot is hardly possible. All we can do is to watch and see what will happen.'[1]

Many doctors were, however, unwilling to merely 'watch and see' whether their patients would develop a deadly disease, and attempted to treat uterine lesions, especially those that were visible during a physical examination of the patient. From Antiquity onwards, doctors applied drugs to uterine tumours, or rather to lesions suspected to be such tumours. In the seventeenth and eighteenth centuries these mixtures were often poisonous substances—for example belladonna, hemlock, strychnine, and lead—applied with the hope of counteracting the 'cancerous poison' with other toxins. Lead-containing ointments were seen as an especially efficient treatment of uterine malignancies. They were credited with the capacity to arrest the tumour's growth and change vaginal secretions into 'laudable pus', a sign of healing. Some doctors, such as Ambroise Paré and the Dutch doctor Herman Boerhaave (1668–1738), treated cervical lesions with milder substances such as rose oil, and juices of pomegranate, leek, and lettuce. However, the majority of their colleagues favoured toxic compounds, especially lead and mercury. The use of the latter substance in treatment of cancerous changes of the cervix was probably linked with its application as a therapy for venereal diseases: in both cases doctors attempted to cure cervical lesions or ulcers.

One of the first images of an extended tumour of the cervix was published in 1793 by the Scottish pathologist Matthew Baillie (1761–1818). The publication of these images may be seen as the beginning of a distinct history of cancer of the womb. Another important turning point was the increase in the use of the speculum. These developments were linked to the rise of gynaecology as a distinct medical specialty. The French surgeon and gynaecologist Joseph Claude Anthelme Récamier (1774–1852) was credited with making the speculum popular again. The Roman and Renaissance speculum was a three-pronged iron instrument employed to dilate the vagina in order to examine the cervix. The insertion of such an instrument was undoubtedly painful, and the visibility it offered was limited. Récamier developed an entirely different kind of instrument: a thin cylinder made of tin, at first straight and later conical. The new speculum had several advantages: it was smooth, allowing for a relatively painless insertion; the tin reflected light, making direct observation easier; and the conical design also improved visibility. Joseph Récamier used the speculum to treat cervical ulcers. His first patient suffered from uncontrollable vaginal discharge. Thanks to the use of a speculum he was able to see clearly ulcerations of the cervix. He then employed the same instrument to apply drugs directly to the observed ulcerations.

Récamier's instrument and its later variants, such as the so-called duckbill speculum developed by the US gynaecologist James Marion Sims (1813–1883) in 1845, greatly improved doctors' capacity to examine the uterine cervix. In the first half of the nineteenth century, the main goal of such examination of the cervix was to detect venereal diseases in prostitutes. In 1810, new police rules in Paris declared that all the registered prostitutes—the only ones allowed to exercise their trade—had to undergo regular gynaecological examinations with a speculum. Such rules were later established in other cities and countries. At that time, the main sign of a venereal disease was ulcerations of external genital organs, the vagina, and the uterine cervix. Women who did not have such ulcerations were declared 'healthy', and were not considered dangerous to their clients. Prostitutes who had visible lesions on their genital organs were obliged to undergo a compulsory treatment in special 'lock hospitals', which often were prison-like structures. They stayed in these hospitals until their doctors declared them 'cured'; that is, free from visible signs of sickness.

The speculum became one of the main symbols of the power of male doctors over a woman's body. Midwives, earlier often entrusted with the task of physical examination of reproductive organs of women, were not allowed to use this instrument. Through its close association with the diagnosis of syphilis and gonorrhoea, the speculum became linked with deviant sexual behaviour. Examination of 'honest' women with a speculum was recommended only in exceptional cases, and some nineteenth-century doctors rejected it altogether. On the other hand, the speculum became a powerful research tool. The compulsory examination of prostitutes provided doctors with rich clinical material. In his study of prostitution in Paris, published in 1836, the French hygienist Alexandre Parent Duchatelet (1790–1836) provided detailed descriptions of periodic examinations of registered prostitutes. Such examinations were often conducted before an audience of medical students and foreign visitors, and one of their goals was to teach the observers how to distinguish between different kinds of uterine lesion. Occasional examinations of 'honest' women with gynaecological complaints provided additional opportunity to learn more about the symptoms of gynaecological diseases. The introduction of the speculum, the US gynaecologist W.O. Baldwin explained in 1884,

> has been to diseases of the womb what the printing press is to civilization, what the compass is to the mariner, what steam is to navigation, what the telescope is to astronomy.... Gynaecology today would not deserve the name of a separate and critical science, but for the light which [the] speculum...has thrown upon it.[2]

The use of the speculum by gynaecologists, sometimes combined with data obtained from the dissection of cadavers, opened the way to studies of pathological changes in female reproductive organs. Doctors occasionally observed 'cauliflower growths'—polyp-like structures that extruded from the cervical wall—and noted that some women with such growths later developed typical syndromes of advanced cancer of the womb. On the other hand, many patients with advanced uterine cancer did not have such polyp-like structures. Some physicians arrived at the conclusion that other lesions of the vulva and the cervix could also degenerate and became cancerous. The accumulation of visual evidence facilitated speculations about links between different kinds of 'cervical sores' and cancer of the womb.

Nineteenth-century theories on origins of cancer of the womb

Two contrasting views of cancer co-existed in the nineteenth century. According to the first, cancer was a systemic disease (it developed at the same time in many parts of the body) rooted in a hereditary predisposition (cancer diathesis). According to the second view, this disease always started as a local lesion which only in its second stage spread to other parts of the body. Cancer, advocates of the latter view argued, was 'a specific and always local irritation of a given organ'.[3] The French doctor Auguste Rossignol explained in 1806 that 'the majority of the experts agree that the cancerous virus is produced at the site of development of this disease, and infects the whole system only when it is carried through the circulation.'[4] The 'local-to-general' hypothesis assumed a continuity between a local 'sore' and a full-fledged cancer. It also assumed that treatment of such a local lesion could prevent the development of a malignant tumour. The latter view, already present in early nineteenth century, was the first version of the slogan diligently promoted by many cancer experts and cancer organizations in the twentieth century: cancer can be cured if treated early.

The local-to-general theory of the origins of cancer was grounded in clinical observations. Physicians had noticed that some malignant tumours, such as cancers of skin, head and mouth, and the breast, started as a local change which gradually increased in size. The term 'cancer' originated from a description of the crab-like spread of malignant tumours of the breast. The development of the cellular theory of cancer in the second half of the nineteenth century consolidated the view that cancer always starts as a local lesion. A new understanding of malignant tumours as an abnormal proliferation of cells provided a plausible explanation of the local-to-general pattern of diffusion of cancerous growths. The spread of cancer, the new theory postulated, was the result of the migration of cancerous cells. The new view of cancer favoured the extension of observation made in a few 'accessible' cancers, such as skin or breast, to all the malignant growths. It was not, however, a necessary condition to the rise of a local-to-general view of cancer. The belief that all cancer had local origins was associated with doctors' attempts to prevent or cure cancer through the elimination of 'sores', 'polyps', or ulcerations that may become cancerous. As the British gynaecologist Robert Barnes put it in 1857,

> The tendency of modern pathologist[s] has been to regard all cancer as local in its origins...this [is] a most hope inspiring doctrine; one to which the clinical physician should cling as that which most encourages therapeutic research and which

alone holds out a prospect of ultimate triumph over the disease.[5]

Nineteenth-century textbooks describe numerous 'sores' of the uterine cervix. Women suffered from granulations in groups, mucous tubercles, scirrhous or scrofulous lesions, projecting spots, superficial ulcerations, corroding ulcerations, engorgement, abrasions, fleshy pimples, vegetations, erosions, and fungous tumours. These lesions were identified by touch, observed using a speculum, and occasionally demonstrated when dissecting a cadaver. One of the main arguments for treatment of all the uterine 'sores' was the hope of preventing malignancy. Cancer, many nineteenth-century physicians believed, started as a reversible 'scirrhous' (indurations or tumefaction); that is, an inflammatory lesion. Later a scirrhous became a 'hidden cancer', more difficult to eliminate, and in its ultimate stages, an incurable, disseminated 'tumour'. It was easy to diagnose the later stages of cancer, but not the earlier ones. The British gynaecologist Edward Rigby stated in 1857 that,

> an accurate diagnosis of this disease in its early stages would indeed be most desirable, but from the nature of it, and of the organ it involves, a medical man has seldom opportunity of examining it at this period, and even if he has, symptoms are at best of an obscure and doubtful character.[6]

As long as unmistaken symptoms of an advanced cancer—uncontrollable blood loss, foul-smelling secretions, severe pain, increase in the volume and hardening of the uterus, and development of tumours in other parts of the body—did not appear, it was difficult to make a firm diagnosis of malignancy. Doctors were therefore strongly advised to refrain from mentioning the word 'cancer' to women with suspicious gynaecological symptoms. Moreover, even if a woman had a cancerous 'sore', doctors hoped to be able to prevent the transformation of a potentially curable scirrhous into an incurable cancer of the womb. Nineteenth-century gynaecologists had conflicting definitions of the point at which a scirrhous was transformed into a 'true' cancer. For some, such a change took place only when the tumour greatly increased in volume, became painful, and developed multiple blood vessels that nourished it. For others, it took place earlier, before the appearance of unmistakable symptoms of an advanced tumour. Even those who held the latter view often believed that an early scirrhous could still be cured.[7] Gynaecologists were aware of the fact that sometimes a fully fledged cancerous growth seemed to appear from nowhere. In the majority of the cases they thought that early warning signs nevertheless made an efficient intervention possible.

The difficulty of providing a precise diagnosis in the early stages of cancer of the womb gave hope to women and their doctors. Women did not know that they had a deadly disease until they presented unmistakable signs of an advanced malignant tumour. Physicians were persuaded that the treatment of suspicious growths, indurations, swellings, abcesses, and chronic irritation of the womb prevented, in some cases at least, the development of a fully fledged cancer. The French gynaecologist Pierre Téalier advised his colleagues to pay attention to all the gynaecological symptoms, however slight, seek their cause, and employ all the tools of their art to eliminate them and avert their return. Writing in 1836, a period of political and social unrest in France, he explained that,

> one often prevents a development which may lead to the dissolution of the social body through an efficient repression of its first movements. Similarly, one can arrest a cancerous

diathesis which, through its progress, invades the whole organism, if one efficiently represses its local symptoms, immediately when they appear.[8]

Control of women's reproductive organs through local application of drugs, intravaginal douches, blood-letting, purging, abstemious diet, and rest could, numerous nineteenth-century doctors believed, keep at bay cancer of the womb, 'this new and wild, unconstrained, uncontrolled form of life'.[9]

Local remedies: corrosive substances, hot iron, and sharp instruments

In the nineteenth century doctors proposed multiple treatments of cervical lesions and uterine tumours. Some treatments were relatively innocuous. Joseph Récamier favoured the therapy already used by Ambroise Paré and Herman Boerhaave: a direct application of fruit extracts such as rose petal syrup. Such extracts, he argued, soothed a sore throat, and could therefore help to heal cervical ulcers as well. Later Récamier also applied to cervical ulcers opium-based preparations such as laudanum, a popular alcoholic herbal preparation which contained approximately 10% opium and 1% morphine:

> I owe to these dressings the amelioration of all the ulcers of the uterus and vagina to which they were applied, the prolongation of lives of several women afflicted with uterine and vaginal cancers, and finally the cure of diverse obstinate ulcerations which were not cancerous.[10]

Other treatments of lesions of the vagina and the cervix were more drastic. Physicians employed caustic substances and cauterization with a red-hot iron, and scraped the damaged tissues with sharp instruments (curettage). Such 'vigorous' therapies were not reserved only for the treatment of suspected cancerous lesions. They were employed in a wide range of gynaecological complaints. In the nineteenth century the uterus was seen as controlling all the female diseases, and stimulation of this organ was perceived as a possible cure for these diseases. Hysteria was related to 'engorgement of the uterus' and the tenderness of the uterine cervix, and doctors sometimes applied corrosive substances to the uterus to cure women's 'nervous conditions'.

The use of strong caustics in the absence of the physical manifestations of disease was probably rare. Corrosive substances were, however, often applied as a therapy for visible lesions of the cervix, especially those suspected to be cancerous. In order to eliminate diseased tissues, physicians employed arsenical paste, hydrate of potassium, nitrate of silver, nitrate of mercury, nitrate of creosote, and potash. Such treatment aimed to cure a less-advanced cancer, and alleviate the symptoms of advanced cancer of the uterus. Physicians employed the speculum to apply corrosive substances directly to cervical lesions. Cauterization was extremely painful. It was nevertheless popular, because physicians believed that once the initial pain subsided a woman obtained relief from the distressing manifestations of her disease: uncontrollable blood loss and repulsive, smelly discharge. Moreover, this treatment reflected the prevailing understanding of the natural history of malignant tumours of the womb. Such tumours were seen as a consequence of poorly controlled inflammation (the term 'tumour' described tumefaction attributed to inflammation), and doctors believed that cauterization would create more active and better-defined inflammation, and would drive the organism to heal both.

The introduction of anaesthesia in the mid nineteenth century made the cauterization itself more bearable. The aftermath of the therapy was, however, harsh. Moreover, some physicians advocated a prolonged application of caustic substances such as Conquin's paste (solid chloral of zinc mixed with flour) to cervical lesions. A French doctor, Bernard Lejeune, wrote in the late 1870 a chilling account of such treatment. Lejeune placed the caustic substance directly on treated cervical lesions and left it there for 24 hours. The treatment was repeated 5 times, to eliminate all the diseased tissue. It produced 'horrid dyspnoea, atrocious pain, only partly alleviated by morphine, convulsions, frissons, fever, severe diarrhoea'.[11] Nevertheless, Lejeune believed that the suffering produced by this procedure was not a sufficient reason for the rejection of a useful therapeutic method.

In the second half of the nineteenth century some physicians attempted to modernize cauterization, and replaced the use of hot irons and caustic substances with destruction of diseased tissues with a galvanic current. Other gynaecologists combined several methods of elimination of diseased uterine tissue: chemical, physical, and mechanical. The latter sometimes included the use of the physician's bare hands. The French gynaecologist François Vuillet explained in 1886 that he first scraped the diseased tissue with a curette and then with his nails. He terminated the treatment with the application of a corrosive substance. William Goodell from Philadelphia proposed in 1880 an inverse order of intervention. He started with cauterization by either hot iron or fuming nitric acid. The diseased tissues were then eliminated with hot wire and battery, cold wire, or spoon curette and scissors, and, if necessary, were finally scraped by hand. Goodell reported that, on one occasion, while scraping away a cancer of the cervix with nails of two fingers, I suddenly found them in the Douglas pouch. I took a good care not to use any vaginal injections, and no undesirable symptoms arose. The patient indeed kept to bed only few days, and then felt good enough to take a long journey home by rail.[12]

'A fate worse than death': the plight of women with uterine tumours

Doctors' willingness to apply harsh treatments to prevent or cure cervical tumours was rooted in their first-hand experience with the disease. Auguste Rossignol, author of an 1806 study of uterine tumours, explained that he decided to study this subject because his sister had died from a uterine cancer: 'her death, preceded by most horrible suffering, left me with a feeling of deep sadness and superfluous regret'.[13]

Many advanced cancers produced distressing symptoms, but women with cervical tumours were especially unlucky. The disease was often very painful, and it frequently progressed slowly. Numerous women lived 1–2 years after their diagnosis (that is, the appearance of symptoms of an advanced cancer), and some lived for several years. Like many people with disseminated cancer, they suffered from general weakness, 'wasting', and pain which was sometimes impossible to control even with high doses of opiates. In addition, however, many women with cancer of the womb suffered from violent and frightening haemorrhages and discharged foul-smelling secretions. The latter symptom occasionally led to social isolation of sufferers and increased their despair. Doctors proposed local treatments to reduce offensive odours of vaginal secretions, such as douching with astringent or deodorizing lotions and tampons and pessaries imbibed with such lotions. They employed alum, ergot, chlorine compounds (chlorates of lime, zinc, iron, and potash), thymol, carbolic acid, and tincture of iodine. Alas, the efficacy of these treatments was often not very high.

In the most dramatic cases, a gradual destruction of internal organs led to formation of a fistula; that is, a permanent connection between the vagina and the urethra and/or rectum. Women with the latter complication of cancer became chronically incontinent, another element that increased their distress and social isolation. A French doctor, Narcisse Mury, described in 1826 women with a fistula that transformed these parts of the body into an 'abominable cloacae, through which women lose blood, urine and faeces'. These unhappy women, Mury added, remain conscious until the end, and were fully aware of their degradation, 'a fate worse than death'.[14]

Some doctors, moved by the extent of suffering of women with uterine tumours, were willing to apply extreme therapeutic means. Other doctors had the opposite reaction: they were not sure whether their efforts to prolong the lives of women with this disease were justified. The French surgeon, anatomist, and pioneer of physical anthropology Paul Brocca (1824–1880) explained in 1866 that cauterization of an ulcerated cervix may stop violent haemorrhages that appear in the late stages of cancer and may give the patient a few additional months of life. He added,

> one may wonder if we are providing a true service to our patients by prolonging a life of suffering and despair, but this is a question a surgeon should not ask. His duty is not to reflect on life, but to fight death.[15]

Women with advanced tumours of the uterus were sometimes abandoned by their own families; they were also frequently rejected by traditional charitable organizations. In France, a pious young widow from Lyons, Jeanne Françoise Garnier-Chabot, founded in 1842 an organization, *L' Association des dames du Calvaire* (the Association of the Ladies of Calvary), that opened hospices for women with advanced uterine cancers. Members of *L'Association*, pious Catholic widows, viewed patients with especially repulsive diseases, such as advanced stages of a disseminated cancer of the womb, as modern equivalents of medieval lepers. Ladies of Calvary washed these women, changed their dressings, and attended to their daily needs, persuaded that overcoming their disgust while doing these tasks allowed them to be closer to Christ. The leaking, disintegrating, decaying, uncontrollable bodies of women in late stages of uterine malignancies became an important site of display of Christian virtues. In the nineteenth century they also became key site for the development of new, daring, and—for some—desperate surgical techniques.

2

SURGICAL CURES FOR A CANCEROUS UTERUS

Desperate surgeons and heroic operations

In 1851, Ada Lovelace's physician, Dr John Locock, examined her internally (probably by touch only, because at that time the speculum was employed nearly exclusively by gynaecologists), diagnosed, 'an extensive and deep seated sore' in her genital organs, and recommended diet, rest, blood-letting, and a liberal supply of pain-killing drugs. Other physicians, we have seen, were more proactive, and attempted to eliminate such sores with cauterization, corrosive substances, or curettage. Others still, especially in France and Germany, proposed an even more radical solution: surgical excision of the cervix and, in rare cases, of the whole uterus (hysterectomy). The latter was an especially dangerous operation that was proposed to women with a pro-lapsed uterus (a uterus that is no longer attached firmly to the abdominal walls), a condition which facilitated the extirpation of this organ. Joseph Récamier excised in 1825 the prolapsed uterus of a 60-year-old woman. The patient survived the opera-tion, and was reported to be alive 3 months later. A Montpelier surgeon, Jacques Mathieu Delpech, became interested in this operation. In 1830 he developed a new technique of surgical excision of the cancerous uterus, and tried it on 21 women, all of whom died.

A less drastic operation, surgical ablation of the cervix, was first proposed by a German surgeon, Johann Frederic Osiander (1787–1855) in 1811. In the 1810s this operation was adopted by Joseph Récamier and other French surgeons. It became less popular in France in the early 1820s, perhaps because of the very high death rate. However, from 1825 onwards it was energetically advocated by a French surgeon, Jacques Lisfranc (1790–1847) from the Parisian hospital Hôtel Dieu. Surgical ablation of the cervix was a truly 'heroic' operation. The surgeon had to employ considerable physical force, while in years before anaesthesia the patient suffered greatly during the surgery itself and in its aftermath. Moreover, the majority of the women operated on died from blood loss and infection. Those who stayed alive after the operation itself were prescribed hot baths, bleedings, enemas, and a severe diet, a post-surgery regime that might have increased mortality rates. Nevertheless, Jacques Lisfranc and his followers claimed that they cured patients who had cancer of the womb. Those who survived the operation led a normal life and one woman who underwent a partial amputation of the cervix even became pregnant.

Other surgeons, appalled by the disastrous outcome of Jacques Lisfranc's operations, contested his optimistic claims. One of Lisfranc's ex-students, Jean Hippolyte Pauly (1806–1854), wrote in 1835 that the majority of women operated at the Hôtel Dieu hospital died from the surgery itself. Those who survived, failed to be cured. Their cancer returned promptly and they died a few months later from their disease. Only one operated patient was still well a year after her surgery, but Pauly did not believe that she had a cancer. One should recall that in the 1820s and 1830s doctors had no certain way of distinguishing the beginning of cancer of the womb from other gynaecological ailments. The most damaging accusation against Lisfranc was that his operation might have killed women who suffered from non-lethal diseases. Lisfranc did not deny that some of his patients did not have a 'true' (that is, advanced) cancer, but said that they had uterine disorders that resisted all treatment. Such untreatable disorders, he argued, nearly always spread beyond the cervix and became disseminated tumours. For these women, the amputation of the cervix was therefore an efficient preventive therapy.

In the 1830s and 1840s, Jacques Lisfranc continued to defend his therapeutic approach, but poor survival rates, coupled with a growing criticism from his colleagues in France and abroad, probably dampened his enthusiasm for surgical ablation of the cervix. He greatly diminished the frequency of these operations in the late 1820s, and quietly abandoned them in the mid 1830s. Between the 1830s and the 1870s the great majority of specialists believed that surgery for cancer of the womb was dangerous and inefficient. Such surgery, mid nineteenth-century gynaecological textbooks explained, only increased the suffering of the unhappy women diagnosed with a malignant tumour. Nevertheless, attempts at surgical cures of cancer of the womb might have influenced nineteenth century medical practice. Claims that the excision of the diseased cervix sometimes—even if rarely—cured cancer of the womb, could had strengthened a view of cancer as a local disease, curable in its early stages. Such claims might have thus encouraged efforts to treat 'predisposing conditions' that led to the development of a fully fledged cancer with drugs or cauterization. Moreover, physicians were aware of the fact that attempts at a surgical excision of a cancerous cervix failed because abdominal surgery was a high-risk enterprise. The development of new approaches that made such surgery safer led to a revival of the aspiration to develop a surgical cure for cancer of the womb.

Radical surgical solutions in the late nineteenth century

The 1870s and 1880s were a period of rapid expansion of surgery. The development of anaesthesia and antisepsis, then of asepsis, encouraged surgeons to attempt more daring surgical operations. The success of some types of abdominal surgery, such as appendicitis, and of gynaecological operations, such as ablation of the ovaries, renewed the interest in surgical approaches to the cure of uterine tumours. At first surgeons' efforts were focused on amputation of the cervix. In the 1870s the German gynaecologist Karl Schroeder (1838–1887) recommended a 'high' amputation of the cancerous cervix; that is, elimination of the cervix together with the lower part of the uterus. Between a third and a quarter of the operated patients died, a result which, while not very good, was decidedly better than those obtained by Lisfranc and his colleagues half a century earlier.

In 1878, another German surgeon who worked in Breslau, Wilhelm Alexander Freund (1833–1917), successfully extirpated a cancerous uterus through the abdominal wall (abdominal hysterectomy). His first results were not very encouraging: 63 of his first 93 patients died following this surgery. The Austrian surgeon Frederich Schauta (1849–1919) proposed in 1891 a somewhat less dangerous surgical technique: the excision of the uterus through the vagina (vaginal hysterectomy). In the 1890s

surgeons estimated that direct mortality from the latter operation was similar to that from a surgical ablation of the cervix:
approximately a quarter of the women operated on died. Many
surgeons were persuaded that more extensive surgery gave the
patient better chances of a cure, and replaced excision of the
cancerous cervix with ablation of the whole uterus.

In the last decade of the nineteenth century, many women
survived hysterectomy for uterine malignancies, but only a
few achieved long-lasting remission. In the great majority of
operated patients, the cancer returned promptly. In spite of
the paucity of long-term cures, surgeons continued to perform hysterectomies. One possible reason might have been a
hope that some women would be saved from an unavoidable
death. Another and perhaps more powerful reason might have
been the observation that women who underwent ablation of
the uterus escaped some of the more distressing symptoms of
advanced malignancy: 'in the majority of cases in which recurrence took place, there was a marked freedom from the fetor
and haemorrhage which are usually so distressing during the
last months of uterine cancer.'[1] Still another element was surgeons' faith in their capacity to improve their techniques. The
French gynaecologist Gustave Richelot recognized in 1894 that
it was not yet possible to know whether hysterectomy could
cure a malignant tumour of the uterus. He performed this operation on 44 cancer patients, and only 2 among them survived for
more than 2 years. Nevertheless, he believed that it was important to continue to perform this operation because 'it is the
most efficient way to find out methods that will bring us closer
to a cure, and will give our patients the longest possible survival
time.'[2] The US gynaecologist Charles P. Noble expressed a similar hope in 1892. The long-term results of hysterectomy were

disappointing,'yet this is probably only a temporary fact, to be disproved by further experience.'[3]

The views of Richelot and Noble were shared by many of their colleagues. At the end of the nineteenth century textbooks of gynaecology stressed that all the women with operable cancers—that is, tumours limited to the uterus—should undergo hysterectomy. Local treatments, such as cauterization or the application of antiseptic substances, once seen as an efficient treatment for an early scirrhous, were redefined as preparatory steps for a surgery or, alternatively, a palliative treatment which could alleviate some of the more bothersome symptoms of women with 'inoperable' cancer; that is, a tumour which had spread beyond the uterus. On 23 October 1899 the French Academy of Medicine organized a debate on treating cancer of the womb. Only one participant in this debate, Dr Desprès, openly opposed surgery for this disease, arguing that he did not believe that a surgical operation could cure an aggressive malignant tumour. All the other participants rejected this view. Surgery, they explained, offered a hope of cure, however slim, and reduced distressing symptoms of the disease. Moreover, women with cancer of the womb had little to lose: 'it is far better for the patient to die under the knife than to face the natural and absolute end.'[4]

One of the results of the rise of surgical radicalism was the inversion of the relation between the size of the lesion and the radicality of the cure. In the early nineteenth century doctors believed that small, localized lesions should be treated by conservative means, and more drastic treatments should be reserved for locally disseminated tumours (cancers which had invaded other internal organs were always seen as being beyond doctors' therapeutic reach). With the growing popularity of surgical treatment of cancer of the womb, many experts adopted the opposite principle. They became persuaded that women with localized tumours were the best candidates for radical surgery, because such surgery offered them a real chance of a cure. This principle was summed up in 1893 by the French gynaecologist Samuel Jean Pozzi (1846–1918): 'the narrower the limits of the disease, the wider the operation should be'.[5]

Vaginal versus abdominal operation

In the 1880s a US surgeon from Johns Hopkins Hospital, Baltimore, William Stewart Halsted (1852–1922), developed a new treatment for cancer of the breast: radical mastectomy. This mutilating surgery, which included the excision of the breast, regional lymph nodes, and part of the chest's muscles, became rapidly the standard operation for breast cancer. In the mid 1890s, two surgeons from Johns Hopkins Hospital, John Clerk and Howard Kelly, proposed a more extensive version of Freund's abdominal hysterectomy, which included removal of the uterus, part of the vagina, ovaries, fallopian tubes, and abdominal lymph nodes. This operation had a high death rate, but, Clerk and Kelly believed that it made long-term cures possible.

In 1898 Austrian gynaecologist Ernst Wertheim (1864–1920) elaborated a somewhat different version of radical abdominal hysterectomy. His technique first became popular in German-speaking countries, and then was adopted by surgeons elsewhere. In the early twentieth century surgeons discussed the relative advantages of the two methods of extirpation of the uterus: vaginal hysterectomy (Schauta's operation) and radical abdominal hysterectomy (Wertheim's operation). The majority of French gynaecologists, and some of those in English-speaking countries, were in favour of vaginal hysterectomy. They argued that abdominal hysterectomy had, c.1900, a much higher mortality rate. It also induced more severe complications in women who survived this surgery. The great majority of women who underwent a vaginal ablation of the uterus had an uneventful recovery, while up to a quarter of those who underwent abdominal hysterectomy suffered from severe bladder or gut problems. Advocates of vaginal hysterectomy also affirmed that the abdominal operation did not produce more long-term cures than the vaginal one.

Advocates of radical abdominal hysterectomy strongly disagreed. They argued that only the opening of the abdominal cavity allowed the surgeon to see whether the cancer had spread beyond the uterus and, if this was the case, either to attempt to eliminate all the abnormal tissues or, if the disease was too advanced, to abstain from a useless intervention. Vaginal hysterectomy did not offer these possibilities. They also pointed to the rapid decrease in mortality from the abdominal operation. Ernst Wertheim reported that when he first introduced his technique a quarter of his patients died during or immediately after the operation. Ten years later only one-tenth of his patients died. In addition, abdominal operation greatly reduced the chances of a rapid local recurrence of cancer. When women underwent vaginal hysterectomy, not infrequently their cancer returned in the operation scar, sometimes as soon as several weeks after the surgery. Such a quasi-immediate return of the cancer was rarely seen after the radical operation. Finally, advocates of abdominal hysterectomy rejected their opponents' claims that the more radical operation did not favour long-term survival. The results of this operation were not very good, since only 10–20% of the patients were alive for 5 years or more, but they were decidedly better than the long-term results of vaginal hysterectomy. The main argument in favour of Wertheim's hysterectomy was, however, surgeons' conviction that only an aggressive approach could cure an aggressive tumour. As the French surgeon Joseph Bouvier put it in 1904: 'there is no doubt that a larger operation will lead to better results'.[6]

Cervical cancer under the microscope

Cancer of the womb was known in Antiquity, but the history of cervical cancer starts in the second half of the nineteenth century. Until the middle of that century physicians were unable to differentiate tumours of the uterine cervix from those of the uterine body. When a reliable diagnosis of this malignancy was made only in advanced stages of the disease—that is, when the tumour had already spread into the abdominal cavity—it was very difficult to establish its starting point as the cervix or body of the uterus. The distinction between these two types of cancer of the womb was possible only in 'early' (that is, localized) cases, precisely those in which it was very difficult to make a firm diagnosis of a malignant tumour.

With the development of better microscopes in the first half of the nineteenth century doctors started to systematically study normal and diseased tissues under the microscope. Those who examined cancerous tissues noticed that malignant tumours are composed of cells that look different from those of the tissue in which the tumour had developed. Cancerous cells were less regular and less well organized, and sometimes had an atypical nucleus. In the 1840s, physicians such as the Swiss doctor Herman Lebert claimed that they could recognize typical microscopic images of cancer cells. At first, the majority of their colleagues remained sceptical. For example, the French surgeon Alfred Velpeau (1795–1867) affirmed in his well-known book on cancer of the breast of 1854 that clinical observations made by an experienced practitioner were much more reliable that microscopic studies. However, the view that cancer is a disease of the cell became increasingly popular in the 1860s and 1870s, thanks to studies of pathologists such as Rudolf Virchow (1821–1902) and Carl Tiersch (1822–1895). At first, microscopic observations of cancer cells were made by researchers who studied the natural history of malignant tumours. However, once doctors had learned how to recognize cancer cells under the microscope they began to apply this knowledge to the diagnosis of malignancies. Microscopic diagnosis was especially useful when doctors needed to decide promptly whether a patient with suspected cancer should undergo risky surgery.

Two doctors from the gynaecological clinics of the University of Berlin, Carl Ruge (1846–1926) and Johann Veit (1852–1917), energetically promoted microscopic diagnosis of cancers of the womb. In the late 1870s and early 1880s Ruge and Veit analysed tissues from the clinics of the pioneer of surgical ablation of the uterine cervix, Karl Schroeder. They showed that among 26 women operated for a presumed early carcinoma in Karl Schroeder's clinics in the Charité Hospital, Berlin, only half had a confirmed malignancy. The other half did not need this traumatic and dangerous surgery (at that time, 1 in 4 women who underwent ablation of the cervix died following this operation). Ruge's and Veit's conclusion was that gynaecologists should not operate on women without a prior confirmation of her cancer diagnosis through biopsy. A woman with suspicious symptoms, such as irregular bleeding, should first undergo a clinical examination with a speculum. If physicians saw a cervical lesion, they needed to excise a small part of this lesion and examine it under the microscope. It they suspected a cancer of uterine body, they needed to do the same with cells collected through diagnostic curettage (scraping of the internal lining of the uterus).

Some experts resisted Ruge's and Veit's conclusions. They continued to believe that their clinical experience was more reliable that microscopic observations. The US gynaecologist Edwin Ricketts argued in 1895 that the rapidly growing 'microscopic menagerie', only increased the confusion around diagnosis of cancer of the womb: 'in the diagnosis of this disease, the microscopic aids have been disappointing, and even misleading. Patient[s] with suspicious symptoms should undergo prompt gynaecological examination, and, if suspicions are confirmed, a vaginal hysterectomy.'[7] Others doctors recognized, however, that microscopic diagnosis was a valuable diagnostic tool, especially when they suspected that their patient had an early stage tumour. Surgeons who claimed that they were able to recognize malignancy by touch thanks to variations in the elasticity of tissues, the German physician Frederich Winckel argued in 1890, were frequently mistaken, because such differences are far from being consistent: 'it is evident from the pathology of carcinoma that in its earlier stages it can be recognized only by the aid of the microscope; this will reveal the characteristic epithelial proliferation of tissues and the consequent destruction of the latter.'[8]

Another use of microscopic diagnosis was to prove the efficacy of therapy. Surgeons who claimed that as many as a third of their patients who underwent radical hysterectomy for uterine cancer were alive and well 5 years after the surgery attributed their good results to their knowledge and skills. Sceptical colleagues who contested their results argued that many of the presumably 'cured' women suffered in fact from a non-malignant gynaecological ailment. Microscopic diagnosis of cancer helped to settle such controversies. The German gynaecologist Alfred Duhrssen (1862–1933) explained in 1895 that only a microscopic examination could put an end to the objection that if the woman recovered permanently, her disease could not have been a carcinoma, 'an objection which is specially urged by Englishmen against the German statistics'.[9]

In the early twentieth century many leading hospitals adopted the principle of a systematic microscopic diagnosis of malignant tumours of the uterus. They performed biopsies of cervical lesions to find out whether they were malignant, and diagnostic curettages to detect suspected cancerous changes. By consequence, the diagnosis 'cancer of the womb' was increasingly replaced with the more precise terms 'cancer of the uterine cervix' or 'cancer of the uterine body'. The systematic distinction between cancers of the uterine body and those, much more frequent, of the uterine cervix had important practical consequences. Before the generalization of hysterectomy, cancer of the uterine body was seen as a disease which had a worse prognosis than cancer of the cervix. Doctors attempted to cure cervical 'sores' with drugs, pomades, and cauterization, but they had no way to treat a disease located in the uterine cavity. However, once cancers of the womb were treated by hysterectomy, gynaecologists found out that cancers of the uterine body had a lower tendency to spread beyond the uterus itself than those of the cervix. More than a third of the women who underwent hysterectomy for cancer of the uterine body in the late nineteenth century were alive 5 years later.

Cervical cancer—in the late nineteenth century approximately 4 times more frequent than cancer of the uterine body—was more difficult to cure. The great majority of women who underwent ablation of the uterus for cervical malignancy died from a generalized cancer. The US surgeon Thomas Stephen Cullen (1868–1953) reported that only 2 among the 60 patients who underwent hysterectomy for cancer of the cervix at Johns Hopkins Hospital in the 1890s were still alive 5 years after the operation. The British surgeon Arthur Lewers similarly observed that only 2–3% of women operated for cancer of the cervix were disease-free 5 years later. Nevertheless, surgeons hoped to improve these results, especially through earlier detection of cervical cancers: 'if cancer of the uterus, whether of the cervix or of the body, be met in a reasonably early stage, there is a very good prospect that permanent relief will be secured by the operative treatment.'[10]

Female surgeons and radical surgery for uterine cancers

Enthusiasm for radical surgical treatment of uterine malignancies was not limited to male physicians, but was shared by some women doctors too. The US surgeon and gynaecologist Mary Amanda Dixon Jones (1828–1908) became a dedicated advocate of surgical ablation of the uterus. Mary Dixon Jones had an unorthodox career. First trained in general medicine, homeopathy, and hydrotherapy, she retrained as a surgeon in her late 40s. She then founded the Women's Hospital of Brooklyn, specialized in surgical treatment of gynaecological diseases. Mary Dixon Jones was the first US surgeon to perform (in 1888) an ablation of the uterus for fibroids (benign tumours). She was persuaded that hysterectomy was the only acceptable treatment for cervical malignancies. Hysterectomy, she argued, should be proposed to all women with operable tumours, but also to those with advanced cancers, because it can provide efficient palliation. This surgery should also be performed in borderline cases:

> the uterus should be removed on suspicion; where there is a doubt that cannot be solved, the patient should have the benefit of this doubt…. Better remove a few organs with no malignant disease than to leave one cancerous uterus, and a patient with the awful risk of dying from a condition that the surgeon could have remedied.[11]

In late nineteenth-century surgical ablation of female reproductive organs—the ovaries and uterus—were alternatively seen as a 'normal' way to treat women, or a transgressive practice. Women were perceived as more disease-prone than men, and many of their health problems continued to be linked to their reproductive functions. It is also likely that some women might have viewed the loss of their ability to carry children as a welcome relief from the tyranny of repeated, unwanted pregnancies. On the other hand, the 'desexing of women' by surgeons was occasionally viewed as a shady, suspicious practice. It was criticized by some practitioners, but also by women who saw it as a manifestation of cruel and unfeeling attitude of gynaecologists towards women's bodies. The doubtful reputation of gynaecological surgeries, coupled with a high mortality from these surgeries, occasionally produced an explosive mix. In 1889, Mary Dixon Jones was accused of second-degree manslaughter after the death of two of her patients, Ida Hunt and Sarah Bates.

Dixon Jones was acquitted of the manslaughter of Ida Hunt, and the Sarah Bates case did not come to a trial. During the trial, a local newspaper, *The Brooklyn Daily Eagle* published a series of articles that accused her of gratuitous cruelty against her patients, performance of ill-advised surgeries, negligence, and incompetence. Dixon Jones, these articles affirmed, was an ambitious and unscrupulous social climber, and a scalpel eager surgeon. *The Eagle* claimed that she told many of her patients who had only slight gynaecological complaints that they suffered from malignant tumours that needed to be excised promptly. Another, smaller Brooklyn newspaper, *The Citizen*, defended Mary Dixon Jones's surgical activity, and presented her as compassionate doctor, concerned exclusively with her patients' well-being. After her acquittal, Mary Dixon Jones sued *The Brooklyn Daily Eagle* for libel. She lost her trial in 1892, and, by consequence, was obliged to abandon the directorship of her hospital and her surgical practice. She dedicated the last years of her life to fundamental research on gynaecological diseases.

The historian Regina Marantz Sanchez, who studied Mary Dixon Jones's tumultuous career, presented evidence that her patient Ida Hunt was a chronically ill young woman, probably as a consequence of venereal disease acquired from her husband. Her surgery might have been a last-ditch effort to regain her lost health. Some women, Marantz Sanchez argued, sought Dixon Jones's clinics precisely because she advocated radical surgical measures. They did not have to be told by Mary Dixon Jones that an ablation of the ovaries or of the uterus was possible. They already knew it, and some were anxious to have such a surgery. Dixon Jones corroborated and empowered her patients' experience, but in an interesting twist, they underscored and sanctioned her therapies as well: 'this may have been especially true, not only because she was a woman doctor but also because she was a radical surgeon who advocated a quick resort to the knife'.[12]

Surgical ablations of the uterus performed by the British surgeons Louisa Garrett Anderson (1873–1943) and Kate Platt (1876–1940) were less controversial. Louisa Garrett Anderson was the daughter of one of the first British female doctors, Elisabeth Garrett Anderson (1836–1917). Louisa Anderson and her colleague and friend Kate Platt co-directed London's New Hospital for Women, specializing in gynaecological operations. Anderson and Platt strongly advocated radical surgery for uterine tumours, a practice they developed in the last years of nineteenth century, and expanded in the first 10 years of the twentieth century. At that time, renowned institutions systematically provided microscopic diagnosis of cancer before attempting a surgical ablation of the uterus. Anderson and Platt attested that all the women who had undergone a hysterectomy for a uterine tumour at their hospital had a microscopically confirmed disease.

At first, Anderson and Platt favoured vaginal hysterectomy. In the early twentieth century they switched, however, to radical abdominal hysterectomy. The latter surgery, they argued in 1908, was not as dangerous as it was presented (they affirmed that the mortality rate at their hospital was 6.6%) while it provided a much more efficient treatment for cancer of the womb. Among the 29 women who underwent a vaginal hysterectomy for cancer of the uterus at the New Hospital for Women, 12 suffered from a prompt return of the cancer in the vaginal scar. By contrast, Anderson and Platt observed such rapid return of the tumour only in 5 among the 58 women who had an abdominal hysterectomy. The long-term results of abdominal hysterectomy were also more promising. Only 1 among the women who underwent vaginal hysterectomy at the New Hospital for Women was alive 5 years after the operation.

The results of abdominal hysterectomy 'cannot be regarded as good, but they are much better than the tragic results we just quoted': 26 patients were symptom-free 1–4 years after the operation, 17 patients had a recurrence, and 15 could not be traced.[13]

Around 1910 the treatment of uterine tumours changed in several important ways. Radical hysterectomy for cancer of the uterus, while still a dangerous operation, was no longer equated with a high probability of imminent death. There was increasing evidence that this treatment saved lives, especially when the patient was diagnosed with cancer of the uterine body. Cervical cancer was more difficult to cure. Still, the surgeons hoped that the perfection of surgical methods would improve the survival of women with this tumour too. New developments did not come, however, from the progress of surgical techniques, but from an entirely new direction: the rise of radiotherapy for cancer. From the 1910s onwards the treatment of cervical cancer was dominated by rays rather than by the scalpel.

3

THE HOPE OF RAYS

The early days of radiation therapy

X-ray therapy of cancer originated in a chance observation. Wilhelm Roentgen (1845–1923) described X-rays in 1895. Scientists who studied the new rays had quickly noticed that they induced burns and blisters. This accidental finding led to speculations about the possibility of using X-rays to destroy unwanted lesions and growths. The first group of physicians interested by the new technique were dermatologists. By 1903 they had developed a long list of conditions that responded favourably to X-ray radiation, from acne to skin cancer. Biologists who studied effects of radiation on tissues had shown that it destroyed rapidly multiplying cells and, for this reason, killed cancer cells selectively. The treatment was not entirely specific. X-rays harmed normal tissues too, especially those rich in rapidly dividing cells: such as bone marrow, the lining of the intestine, and hair roots. Such destruction of normal tissues produced the distressing side effects of X-ray therapy: anaemia, digestive disorders such as diarrhoea and nausea, and hair loss.

With the discovery of radium by Pierre Curie (1859–1906) and Marie Curie-Sklodowska (1867–1934) in 1898, physicians had found a second source of radiation with potential medical applications. The therapeutic applications of radium also stemmed from a chance observation. In 1901 the French co-discoverer of radioactivity, Henri Becquerel (1852–1908), had noticed that radium produced burns (according to one story, he carried a tube of radium in his watch pocket and discovered that he developed a burn on his chest). This observation was rapidly followed by experiments using the new source of radiation to treat skin diseases and cancerous growths. Scientists had found that therapeutic effects of radium were akin—although not identical—to those of X-rays. Radiation therapy also produced similar side effects. The main difference was that, unlike X-rays, radiation produced by radium acted only at close distance. During the early years of development of radiation therapy, a radium source, often enclosed in thin glass or metal tubes, was placed in the immediate vicinity of the treated lesion (brachytherapy). In the 1920s, thanks to the discovery of rich mines of uranium in the Belgian Congo, the radium industry was able to supply greater quantities of this element. It then became possible to use powerful sources of radium (radium bombs) for treatment at a distance (teletherapy). This new use of radiation therapy was sometimes combined with a proximity treatment. Some tumours responded better to X-rays, and others to various forms of radiation therapy. In the interwar era all three approaches—X-rays, radium needles, and radium bombs—were applied successfully to the treatment of cervical cancer.

X-rays and then radium were rapidly employed to treat skin cancer and gynaecological malignancies. The American gynaecologist Barton Cooke Hirst mentioned in 1903 the use of

'Roentgen and Fissen rays' to treat tumours of the womb. He explained that 'it is too early to decide what the ultimate results of the X-ray treatment of cancer of the cervix will be. A cure can hardly be expected, but there is no doubt of the enormous relief afforded. Haemorrhage often ceases, the discharge diminishes or disappears, and a patient practically bedridden may be restored to an active life'.[1] A 1904 book on the use of radiation in the treatment of cancer noted that it was difficult to use this therapy for internal tumours, but, 'in pelvic carcinomata the results have been somewhat better, mainly because it has been possible to bring the source of the rays into closer contact with the tumour by making use of the vagina'.[2] The same year a New York physician, Dr Robert Abbe, experimented with intravaginal applications of radium. Other doctors confirmed that radiation therapy could be applied to the treatment of uterine growths. The new therapy was reported to be efficient in reducing pain and odour. Doctors witnessed a quasi-miraculous shrinking of extended, ulcerated cervical tumours and a marked improvement of distressing symptoms of advanced cancer. Radiation therapy of advanced uterine tumours changed the image of this disease. The US radiation specialist Daniel Quigley explained in 1929 that thanks to new therapeutic approaches 'we have been able to uncover the fact that something exists in cancer besides the terminal, fatal, bleeding, painful, stinking stage'.[3]

The first institution dedicated to therapeutic applications of radium was Laboratoire Biologique du Radium in Paris. It was founded in 1906 by Armet de Lisle, owner of a radium factory and collaborator of Pierre and Marie Curie. De Lisle's initiative was not exceptional. In the early twentieth century producers of radium, often people with scientific training and interests, frequently collaborated with leading physicists, and often played an important role in the development of medical applications of the new substance. The physicians who worked at the Laboratoire Biologique du Radium—Pierre Degrais, Louis Wickham, and Henri Domenici—came from the Saint Louis Hospital, Paris, specialized in the treatment of skin diseases, and at first applied radium as a therapy for dermatological disorders. Research at the Laboratoire Biologique du Radium rapidly turned, however, to the application of radium in treating other diseases, among them gynaecological ailments.

In 1908 Henri Domenici developed a thin, sealed metal tube which allowed only gamma radiation—the rays that selectively harmed cancer cells—to pass through it (the filtration method). He then used his tubes to treat cancer of the uterus, and found out that the results were decidedly better than those obtained with non-filtered radiation. In 1912 Domenici was named head of the radiation therapy department at the Rothschild Hospital, Paris. The hospital was founded by the industrialist Henri de Rothschild, another pioneer of the radium industry in France (his factory, Société Anonyme des Traitements Chimiques, produced instruments for medical application of this element). The same year, radiation therapy departments were opened in hospitals in three additional French cities. The extension of radiation therapy in France was part of a more general trend. The London Radium Institute was founded in 1911. The Institute's physicians also initially specialized in therapy of skin diseases, including skin cancer, then started to treat other 'accessible' cancers. In 1910 physicians who experimented with radiation therapy noticed that some tumours reacted well to radiation therapy, while others were less affected by rays. Breast cancer, they and other experts had found, was relatively radioresistant. By contrast, cervical cancer was highly radiosensitive, and was a very good candidate for radiation therapy.

Radiation therapy dramatically changed the treatment of cervical tumours. Between 1890 and 1910 specialists gradually adopted radical hysterectomy as the state-of-the-art treatment of cervical cancer. This was, however, a problematic cure. The surgery itself was dangerous, with an average 10–15% immediate mortality, while even in the best centres only about a third of the women who survived radical hysterectomy were alive and symptom-free 5 years or more after their operation. X-ray or radiation therapy offered an attractive alternative to surgical ablation of the uterus. The main advantage of this treatment was its lower mortality. Radiation therapy was not, to be sure, totally risk-free. The most frequent severe complication was infection. When the cancerous lesion was infected by pathogenic bacteria radiation treatment could lead to a generalized abdominal sepsis, nearly always fatal in the pre-antibiotics era. In spite of this danger, the rate of mortality from radiation therapy—2–4%— was much lower than that from radical hysterectomy.

An additional advantage of radiation therapy of cervical cancer was that it usually did not induce prolonged invalidity. When doctors employed an external source of radiation the treatment was often conducted on an outpatient basis. Women treated internally with radium needles or tubes had to be hospitalized for the duration of their treatment, but if everything went well they could rapidly return to their usual occupations. By contrast, women who underwent a radical hysterectomy remained incapacitated for weeks and sometimes for months after the surgery, a serious practical problem for those with a job or young children and who could not afford domestic help. Some women systematically denied severe gynaecological symptoms because they were afraid of surgery and its consequences. Therefore they missed a chance to be cured. When the proposed treatment was less drastic and less dangerous these women could be more easily persuaded to see a doctor. Finally, surgery could not help women with advanced, 'inoperable' cervical cancer, while radiation therapy frequently attenuated distressing symptoms produced by disseminated tumours, and occasionally produced long-lasting remissions in women diagnosed with such tumours. Women who were classified earlier as hopeless cases and were sent home to die were offered treatment, relief, and hope. No wonder that radiation therapy was hailed by the popular press as a miraculous cure for cancer of the womb.

Diffusion of the new technique

In the early days of radiation therapy, this method was occasionally applied by gynaecologists in private practice who purchased a small quantity of radium. More efficient treatments were, however, developed in specialized institutions. In the 1910s two centres played an important role in treatment of cervical tumours by rays: the Radiumhemmet in Stockholm, Sweden, and the Curie Foundation at the Radium Institute (later the Curie Institute) in Paris. Both were charitable institutions which received at the same time governmental support. The Radiumhemmet, founded in 1910 and directed by Gösta Forsell (1876–1950), specialized in treatment of gynaecological cancers. One of the Radiumhemmet's experts, James Heyman (1882–1956), published in 1915 a text on the 'Stockholm method' of radiation therapy of cervical tumours, an approach rapidly adopted by other institutions.

The Radium Institute of Paris, founded thanks to an important private bequest, was inaugurated in 1912. It was linked with two institutions: Marie Curie's laboratory of physics in the Radium Institute was affiliated with the Science Faculty of the University of Paris, and a laboratory in the institute dedicated to studies of the biological effects of radiation was affiliated with the Pasteur Institute. The director of the latter, Emile Roux (1853–1933), named in 1913 Claudius Regaud (1870–1940), a Lyon physician who studied the physiological effects of radiation, as the director of the biology laboratory. Regaud was soon joined by his ex-collaborator from Lyon, Antoine Lacassagne (1884–1971). At first, the new biology laboratory, named 'Pavillon Pasteur', was dedicated to fundamental research on the physiological effects of radiation. Regaud's experience as head of a medical radiology unit during the First World War led him, however, to an interest in the application of radium and X-ray radiation to the treatment of cancer. After the war, Regaud brought to the Radium Institute some of his collaborators at the army's medical radiology unit, among them Henri Coutard (1876–1949), who became the leader of the Institute's school of X-ray therapy.

In 1920, Marie Curie and Claudius Regaud received an important donation from the industrialist Henri de Rothschild for the promotion of therapeutic activities at the Radium Institute. This donation, named the Curie Foundation, enabled the Institute to purchase radium and X-ray equipment and to open a dispensary dedicated to the ambulatory treatment of cancer patients. Physicians who worked at the new dispensary collaborated with biologists and physicists from the Radium Institute, while its directors, Claudius Regaud and Antoine Lacassagne, shared their time between fundamental biological studies at the Pavillon Pasteur and treatment of cancer patients at the dispensary. Close links between the laboratory and the clinics favoured technological innovations such as the improvement of methods of delivery of X-rays, better selection of more penetrating rays produced by radium, and more accurate quantification of the amount of radiation delivered to patients. These innovations increased in turn the efficacy of radiation therapy and reduced its side effects. At first the Curie Foundation specialized in the local application of radium needles, but a gift of 1 g of radium from the American Women's Movement to Marie Curie made possible the development of teletherapy: the treatment of tumours at distance.

Women with cancer of the cervix who received local radiation therapy at the Curie Foundation had to stay in hospital several days. The patient's cervix was first dilated under anaesthesia, then her physicians inserted radium needles or radium seeds in small capillary tubes and packed the cervical cavity with sterile gauze. The patient was kept immobile in bed for a few days, and she was usually given painkillers. The radium was then removed under local or general anaesthesia and the woman was sent home. More affluent patients were hospitalized in private clinics. Charity patients were treated in a special ward opened in 1919 at the Pasteur Institute's Hospital.

In the early 1920s, radiation therapy of 'operable' uterine cancers at the Curie Foundation was systematically combined with hysterectomy. The patient was first treated with radium, then had a surgery. In the mid 1920s the Foundation's physicians arrived at the conclusion that radiotherapy alone—usually a combination of external and local irradiation—was as efficient as the combination of radiotherapy with surgery. The perfection of radiotherapy techniques improved the survival rates of patients with localized cervical cancer; that is, one that was

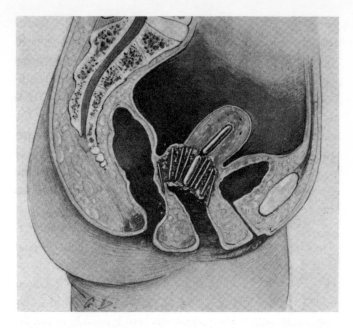

1. Diagram illustrating section in the intrauterine tubes and the disposition of
needles in the modified Stockhom method.

strictly limited to the cervix. In the interwar era, 60–70% of
such patients treated exclusively with rays were alive 5 years
after diagnosis.

Swedish and French institutions became models for cancer-
treatment centres in other Western countries such as the Marie
Curie Hospital in London, the Memorial Hospital in New York,
or the Institut fur Krebsforschung (Institute for Cancer Research)
of the Berlin Charité hospital. The high cost of radium played a
key role in the centralization of radiation therapy. In the 1920s,
the company of the Belgian Mines du Haut-Katanga (Upper

Congo Mines) lent to Marie Curie several grams of radium. Another French centre, the Villejuif Cancer Institute, affiliated with the Medical School of Paris University, received a similar temporary gift. The Stockholm Radiumhemmet was able to purchase radium thanks to a gift of 6 million crowns received in 1928 from King Gustav V (the money was originally a gift of the Swedish people to the king for his seventieth anniversary). In the USA, the engineer James Douglas, co-founder of an important radium production plant in Denver, Colorado, donated his share of the company in the form of several grams of radium to the Memorial Hospital for the Treatment of Cancer and Allied Diseases in New York. In the UK, the Royal Air Force had at the end of the First World War a surplus of 5 g of radium (the element was used to paint the dials of navigation instruments in aeroplanes). It donated this surplus to the Medical Research Council, which in turn loaned it to the Middlesex Hospital in London. In 1929 the British government created the National Radium Commission which supervised the distribution of radium to regional cancer-treatment centres.

Doctors in Germany and Austria resisted in the 1920s and 1930s the use of X-rays and radium to treat women with 'operable' cervical tumours, or those which could be alternatively treated by surgery alone. Such resistance was grounded in the existence of a strong tradition of surgical therapy of uterine tumours (from the late nineteenth century onwards German surgeons claimed to have better long-term results for hysterectomy than their French or English colleagues) and in physicians' opposition to the centralization of cancer treatment in specialized centres. German-speaking countries were exceptional in this regard. In other Western countries, cervical cancer was increasingly treated by rays, often in combination with

other therapeutic approaches. Radiation treatment was sometimes followed by ablation of the uterus, or, inversely, hysterectomy was followed by X-ray radiation; external X-rays were
employed to strengthen the effect of radium needles; women
were treated with combinations of X-rays and radium needles or with radium needles and a radium bomb; radiotherapists collaborated with surgeons to place radiation sources in
the abdominal cavity to irradiate regional lymph nodes. Such
complex therapies were frequently conducted in specialized
centres. In the 1930s the treatment of cervical cancer was one
of the first examples of the constitution of multidisciplinary
teams of doctors who worked together to promote the cure of
a single disease.

Women physicians and radiotherapy of cancer

In the late nineteenth and early twentieth centuries some
women surgeons, such as Mary Dixon Jones or Louisa Garrett
Anderson, embraced the male surgeons' ethics of daring behaviour and willingness to take risks. Their attitude might have
been motivated by an aspiration to demonstrate that, as professionals women physicians are not different from men. Other
women physicians had chosen a different approach. They saw
themselves as spokespersons for their sex, and promoted treatments which, they believed, were less harmful and more acceptable for women.

The radiological treatment of uterine cancer, the British
pioneer of medical statistics statistician Janet Elizabeth Lane-
Claypon (1887–1977) explained, provides similar rates of cures
to surgical treatment without many of its risks, disadvantages,
and inconveniences:

it is clear that one of the most serious deterrents for patients needing early advice and treatment for cancer is the dislike of the operation. If this fear can be removed by substituting another method of treatment, a great impulse might be expected in the movement for securing the attendance of patients at hospital in an earlier stage of their malady.[4]

'Dislike of the operation' was a mild way to describe the reluctance of women with slight symptoms such as irregular bleeding to undergo a surgery that had a 10% chance of killing them, which incapacitated them for several months and put them at risk of chronic digestive or urinary problems. Women with extended tumours were often in a great deal of pain, and were therefore less reluctant to undergo radical surgery. These women were, however, usually classified as 'inoperable'. Radiation therapy had the double advantage of proposing a less traumatic treatment in 'curable' cases, and relief in 'incurable' ones.

In the UK, women played an important role in the development of radiation therapy of gynaecological cancers, above all cancer of the uterine cervix. In 1924 a committee of the Medical Women's Federation (MWF) set up a project to investigate the efficacy of radium in the treatment of cervical cancer. Thanks to the MWF's support, three hospitals staffed by women doctors— the Elisabeth Garrett Anderson Hospital, the South London and New Sussex Hospital, and the Royal Free Hospital—established together a clinic dedicated to radiation therapy of gynaecological cancers. In 1929, this clinic was transformed into a 30-bed hospital, run by women physicians, called the Marie Curie Hospital, situated in London. Cervical cancer was presented by MWF activists, such as Helen Chambers, as a domain where women's medical needs would be best served by female practitioners. The writer Vita Sackville-West (1892–1962) explained in a fund-raising leaflet for the Marie Curie Hospital that this hospital 'ministers to peculiarly feminine ailments, and no one but a woman can know what they mean'. Women were reluctant to talk with male doctors about these ailments. They were relieved when they could go to a hospital where a woman:

> can meet other women who, though doctors, speak the same intimate language as herself; women to whom no revelation is novel, even the most secret fears and shyness and atavistic complexes, then her reluctance [to consult a physician] may be modified and the danger taken before it is too late.

Moreover, Sackville-West added, women from lower social strata often dreaded operations in charity hospitals because they were afraid to be used as experimental material. Radiation therapy did not generate such fears: women knew that 'their poor bodies will not be carved up while they lay under the arc lights unconscious and without defence'.[5]

In Britain, hospitals staffed with women and specializing in radiation therapy opened new professional opportunities for women physicians. This was true in France too, despite the absence of hospitals staffed by women. Several French women physicians became pioneers of radiation therapy of cervical cancer. One the reasons female physicians were attracted to the new domain was career opportunities. In the interwar era women physicians had no chance whatsoever of entering the official career track in the French medical system, of receiving the title of *aggregé de médicine*, of becoming head of department in a university hospital, of being appointed to a university chair. Institutions such as the Curie Foundation in Paris, and the Villejuif Cancer Institute, at the margins of the official system of academic medicine, were more apt to promote women's careers. Several women physicians were trained at the Curie Foundation and later became pioneers of *curitherapy*, the French term for radiation therapy. Among them were Juliette Baud, who directed radiation therapy services at the Curie Foundation, and Simone Laborde, head of the radiation therapy service at the Villejuif cancer centre.

Simone Laborde, a physician married to Pierre Curie's student and close collaborator, Albert Laborde, played an important role in the development of radiation therapy for cervical tumours in France. Laborde was less inclined than some of her colleagues to use 'heroic' therapeutic measures. She contested the principle of a prolonged irradiation of the uterus and the use of high radiation doses. These therapeutic strategies were grounded in the belief that in the 'war against cancer' more is always better. Simone Laborde was not persuaded that this was the case. She did not view malignant tumours as an alien enemy but as a diseased part of the body. The sensitivity of malignant tissues to radiation, Laborde argued, does not depend only on the irradiated cells themselves, but on their interactions with their immediate environment. Destruction of healthy tissues through excessive radiation not only produced more severe side effects, but also reduced the efficacy with which the body could eliminate cancerous tissues. In the 1930s Laborde warned against the false security provided by new, more powerful sources of radiation. While these new sources produced often less visible secondary effects such as burns, the accumulation of their effects still frequently induced severe complications. Simone Laborde's experience persuaded her that more moderated radiation doses were often as efficient as the more elevated ones: 'producing an increasingly extended destruction of cells, will certainly not led us to the solution of the cancer problem'.[6]

Not an entirely benign procedure

Simone Laborde's warnings against the use of excessively high doses of radiation were grounded in her clinical practice. X-ray treatment and radiation therapy, although often less traumatic than Wertheim's radical hysterectomy, were far from being innocuous procedures. The treatment produced numerous undesirable symptoms. Some of these symptoms: skin burns, digestive and urinary problems, nausea, and fatigue, were relatively mild, or at least manageable, if the woman was lucky. Radiation therapy experts affirmed that, in spite of some unavoidable secondary effects, many of their patients were able to continue their daily occupations during their treatment. They took care of their housework and families, and those who had a job kept it. Moreover, in the majority of cases, distressing symptoms disappeared several months after the end of the treatment.

However, in a minority of women radiation therapy produced severe complications and lasting mutilations. One of the worst was a vaginal fistula which led to chronic incontinence. A vaginal fistula was also one of the complications of hysterectomy, and, we have seen, of disseminated cervical cancer. A fistula can sometimes be corrected by surgery, but corrective surgery was more problematic in women who underwent radiation therapy because irradiated tissues often failed to heal properly. Radiation therapy could also produce inflammation, painful thickening or necrosis of the skin, oedema of legs, severe digestive problems, and abdominal, skeletal, and limb pain. The medical historian Barbara Clow quotes a Canadian woman who in the 1930s wrote to the Ontario Department of Health to explain why she had refused radiotherapy for cervical cancer:

> three of my friends had similar treatment and the told me they were dying a death of a fiery infernal furnace. Knowing of their untimely death and awful agony, I was determined to die comfortably, if need be by the inroads of cancerous growth.[7]

Radiotherapy was sometimes as 'heroic' as a radical surgery was. The treatment was often long and debilitating, and some of its severe complications probably made the life of patients no less miserable than the life of those who suffered from complications of radical surgery for cancer. Radiotherapy experts elected to focus on the advantages of the radiation treatment rather than on its drawbacks. Physicians at the Curie Foundation viewed many of the secondary effects of radiotherapy as normal. In many cases, patient records from the 1920s and 1930s contain the global evaluation 'the patient is well' (read: cancer-free) and, at the same time, a long list of the patient's complaints: pain, scarified skin, digestive and urinary problems, insomnia, difficulty in keeping specific positions, and reduced mobility. In some cases letters from cured patients, appended to their files, describe their poor health and chronic suffering.[8] Women physicians at the Marie Curie Hospital in London similarly elected to put to the fore the good results of radiation therapy. The hospital's director, Elisabeth Hurdon, recognized nevertheless that some patients suffered from severe late complications of this therapy, such as blockage of the intestines, injuries to the bladder and the urethra, bone necrosis, and rectal ulcers: 'sometimes the rectal reactions occur several years after the treatment. Patients who were perfectly well start to develop pelvic pain and digestive problems.'[9]

In France and the UK, public health authorities were persuaded that in many cases complications of radiation therapy for cervical tumours were the result of doctors' incompetence. Some gynaecologists in private practice purchased a small amount of radium, and applied it in a haphazard way to the treatment of cervical tumours. Experts such as Claudius Regaud warned against risks of such amateurish treatments, and strongly advocated the concentration of radiation therapy in the hands of well-trained and experienced practitioners. One of the goals of the centralization of cancer treatment in France in the interwar era was to promote better training of radiotherapists and reduce the frequency of therapeutic accidents.

In the 1930s many European countries introduced the centralized regulation of radiation therapy of cancer. At that time such regulation did not yet exist in the USA. In 1937 Maurice Lentz (1890–1974), director of the radiotherapy service at the Presbyterian Hospital in New York City and one of the pioneers of radiation therapy in the USA, was asked by the American Radium Society to conduct a survey about the use of radiation in the treatment of cancer of the cervix. The survey provided a glimpse into the practices of US doctors. Radiation therapy was administered by qualified radiologists who worked in specialized centres, but also by inexperienced physicians who worked in small hospitals or used radium in private practice. Experienced radiologists obtained good results: low levels (2% or less) of treatment-related mortality and moderate rates of severe complications. Doctors who employed radium in private practice or small hospitals reported much higher rates of severe complications. Lentz and his colleagues from the American Radium Society believed that the main culprit was the use of excessively high doses of radiation, and attempted to educate doctors with a view to homogenizing their practices. Some physicians resisted such efforts. Dr Edward Skinner from Kansas City explained that:

I have been handling carcinoma of the cervix for a matter of 20 years and think that my results have been comparatively satisfactory. I have always used very large doses and have never been content with 3000 or 3600 milligram/hour [the dose employed by the great majority of the interrogated physicians]. I even take some of my cases up to 9600 milligrams/hour....I have no statistics for you. I realize that they are necessary for your type of report. I have no income other than that from my patients, no endowment, no tax-support and no angel. I am not connected with a teaching institution other than a dental school. I am not going to burden my patients with any extra expense of statistics. I am no longer interested in the parade of science. I wish you good luck with the standardization committee report. It is more of a job than I would undertake.[10]

Amateurish application of radiation therapy put patients at risk. Alas, careful and well-informed use of radiation did not eliminate all the dangers of this therapy. Radiotherapists faced difficult decisions, especially when they treated locally advanced cervical cancers. A too timid attitude could rob some women of the chances of a cure; an overly aggressive one could produce iatrogenic (doctor-induced) disease. Maurice Lentz's student, Franz Buschke, head of the radiotherapy department at the Tumor Institute of the Swedish Hospital, Seattle, Washington, USA, reported that approximately one quarter of women with locally disseminated cervical cancer who were treated with a combination of radiation therapy and high-voltage X-ray treatment developed a severe inflammation of the rectum. Half of the affected women recovered; the other half developed severe ulceration of the rectum and died from this complication.[11] In women with advanced cervical cancer, miracle cures were, alas, rare.

Buschke made a last-ditch effort to treat women with otherwise incurable cancer. Occasionally radiation therapy of less-advanced, and in principle curable, tumours also produced severe side effects. In some cases doctors were not sure whether the patient suffered from complications of radiation or the return of her cancer. Radiation therapy could produce scarring of internal organs which mimicked distressing symptoms of disseminated cancer of the cervix. Before the era of advanced medical imagery technologies, only exploratory abdominal surgery could tell whether a woman suffered from cancer or the late effects of radiation. Such a surgery was, however, a risky endeavour, the more so because irradiated tissues cicatrized poorly. In the pre-antibiotic era, physicians often elected a wait-and-see approach. If the patient deteriorated, physicians at the Marie Curie Hospital in London explained, her symptoms were interpreted as the return of her cancer and if she got better or remained stable they were seen as complications of radiotherapy.[12]

Physicians at the Curie Foundation in Paris encountered similar diagnostic problems. Some of the women diagnosed with cervical tumours and treated with radiation therapy, X-rays, or both developed several years later symptoms, such as chronic pain, digestive problems, and—in rare cases—a fistula. Such symptoms might have been signs of late complication of radiotherapy, a recurrence of cancer, or a combination of both. Patient's files from the Curie Foundation illustrate the sometimes troubling similarities between description of advanced cervical tumours and complications of treatment of such tumours, numerous diagnostic dilemmas, and the presence of some unresolved cases.[13]

The dramatic fate of patients who suffered from severe complications of radiation therapy may be presented as an

A WOMAN'S DISEASE

argument against the 'burning' of cancer cells with rays. Some women, like the one quoted by Barbara Clow, elected to die from cervical cancer rather than to be exposed to a 'death of a fiery infernal furnace'. One should remember, however, that the main reason for doctors' difficulty in distinguishing between secondary effects of radiotherapy and the spread of cancer was that both produced similar—and similarly harsh—symptoms. It is also important to remember that severe complications of radiotherapy were relatively rare. This treatment alleviated the suffering of many women, and definitively cured some among them. On the other hand, radiotherapy did not fulfil early hopes that it would cure the majority of cervical malignancies. In spite of rapid improvement of radiotherapy methods and the availability of much more powerful radiation sources, on average 4 out of 5 women diagnosed with cervical cancer in the interwar era still died from their disease.

How efficient was the treatment of cervical cancer?

In the 1920s the medical statistician Janet Lane-Claypon studied the efficacy of treatments for breast and cervical cancers. Lane-Claypon had a double training, in medicine and physiology. In the 1910s she became interested in epidemiology and developed a new method of epidemiological investigation, the cohort study. In 1923 the British Minister of Health, Neville Chamberlain, set up a committee to look into causation, prevalence, and treatment of cancer. Janet Lane-Claypon was hired by the ministry to collect data on this subject.[14] Her surveys, conducted with great methodological care, became standard references on the efficacy of cancer therapies. Lane-Claypon was a prominent member of the statistical committee of the Cancer Commission of the League of Nations, and her results were reproduced in the League's publications and in medical journals in numerous countries.

Janet Lane-Claypon's studies pointed to direct relationships between the degree of advancement of a breast tumour and cure rates. Only women with small, localized cancers had a good chance of being alive 5 years after a mastectomy. Lane-Claypon did not speak about 'early' tumours. Her main distinction was between cancers limited to the breast and those which had spread to lymph nodes and beyond. She might have been aware of the possibility that at least some of the 'localized' tumours did not spread beyond the breast because they grew slowly, not because women diagnosed with these tumours had had an early consultation with their doctors. Her findings were, however, presented as a proof of the key role of early detection, were translated into a strong recommendation to consult a doctor immediately upon noticing suspicious symptoms, and were interpreted by some as an implicit supposition that a woman diagnosed with an advanced breast tumour brought her plight upon herself.

Lane-Claypon's survey of the literature on cancer of the cervix indicated that the links between the stage at which a cervical cancer was diagnosed and chances of cure were somewhat more complicated. The disease often produces symptoms only in the more advanced stages. Cancers which extended beyond the uterus at the moment of diagnosis were nearly always fatal, whereas those which were limited to the cervix had a reasonably good prognosis, but many among the newly diagnosed cervical cancers were classified as 'locally advanced tumours'. Some 30–40% of women with such tumours were cured, while the others succumbed to their disease. It was difficult to predict what the fate of a given woman with a locally advanced tumour would be.

Janet Lane-Claypon's analysis of treatment of uterine cancer at the Samaritan Free Hospital, London, confirmed the trends she had deduced from compilation of the medical literature. At that time the Samaritan Free Hospital did not offer routine radiation therapy. Women with 'operable' cancers of the womb underwent hysterectomy, whereas those with 'inoperable' ones received only palliative care. Lane-Claypon studied the files of 1,023 women at the Samaritarian Free Hospital. One-fifth had cancer of the uterine body and the other four-fifths had cancer of the cervix. Fifty-three per cent of the women diagnosed with cervical cancer, and 79% of those diagnosed with cancer of the uterine body, were classified as 'operable'. Among the latter, 35% of women who underwent hysterectomy for cervical cancer, and 60% of those who underwent this operation for cancer of the uterine body, were alive 5 years after the surgery.[15] To sum up, roughly 47% of women diagnosed with cancer of the uterine body, and 18% of those with cancer of the cervix, were cured.

Janet Lane-Claypon was appalled by the high mortality from cervical cancer. She might have also been moved by the plight of women she had seen at the Samaritarian Free Hospital. She concluded that:

> The high number of cases judged inoperable reveals a serious need for the adoption of means to secure earlier attendance at hospital on the part of women suffering from cancer of the cervix. It is not possible at present to assign the responsibility for this disastrous state of affairs, but further investigation is urgently necessary.[16]

An editorial in the British Medical Journal similarly bemoaned, 'the deplorable number of women who delay applying for treatment until [the cancer] is in an inoperable state', and suggested that, 'further efforts should be made to discover and remove the causes of this disastrous delay'.[17]

'Staging' tumours

Cancer experts did not need Janet Lane-Claypon's data to realize that women with localized cancer had a better chance of being cured than those with more extended malignancy. Comparison of results of treatments made sense only if these treatments were applied to women with a similar disease. But was it known that this was the case? Physicians indicated in their publications the proportion of 'localized', 'locally advanced', and 'generalized' tumours among their patients. These were, however, subjective definitions: a cancer classified as localized by one doctor could have been classified as locally advanced by another. The whole domain, Antoine Lacassagne complained in 1922, was highly confused: 'there is no uniform classification of malignant tumours or a universally recognized description of their properties, or even a way to compare different terminologies. A research report may be fully understood only by its author.'[18]

The obvious solution was the homogenization of clinical diagnoses of cancer. Such homogenization was a difficult task, because it relied on the tacit knowledge of the expert. Even doctors who worked together did not always propose identical classification. When Claudius Regaud reviewed Antoine Lacassagne's clinical notes, he pencilled several objections to the diagnosis of stage II cancer (local extension of the tumour) proposed by Lacassagne. His own proposition was that this was either stage I tumour (limited to the cervix) or stage III (extended beyond the uterus):

> case no. 3. Classified as stage II. It looks like a typical stage I cervical epithelioma. But there is also a small node, size of a coffee grain...on the right hand side. This small node was treated by radium therapy at a distance. The nature of this small node was not defined with precision. This is an unusual location for a cancerous lymph node in cervical cancer. If this node should be seen nevertheless as a cancerous lymph node, this a stage III and not stage I cancer. If we do not take it into consideration, this is indeed a stage I—this is my proposal. But there is no place in this case for a stage II.[19]

On the other hand, all the experts agreed that homogenization of diagnoses was the only way to know which treatments worked best. Such a homogenization—the international classification of cervical tumours—was promoted by the Cancer Commission of the League of Nations in the 1920s and 1930s. Members of the Commission of Cancer of the League of Nations appointed a 'classification commission', presided over by James Heyman from Radiumhemmet, Stockholm. The commission's report became the basis of the Heyman international system of classification of cervical tumours. This system defined 4 stages of progression of cervical cancer. In stage I cancers, the growth was strictly limited to the cervix. In stage II, the cancer had spread to the whole uterus. In stage III, cancerous cells infiltrated the ligaments that link the uterus to the pelvic wall, and might have spread to neighbouring lymph nodes. In stage IV, the cancer had spread to organs close to the uterus, and in more advanced cases to remote organs as well. In the 1930s the majority of cancer centres adopted Heyman's international system. In the 1950s the principles which governed the classification of cervical cancers were extended to all malignant tumours. Heyman's system became a model for an international classification of cancers, the TNM system (which stands for Tumour, Lymph Nodes, Metastases); this system is still employed in the early twenty-first century.

Thanks to the introduction of a uniform system of classification of cervical cancers, doctors were able to compare the results of treatments of this disease. They realized then that, in the hands of competent specialists, all the approaches were equally good (or equally disappointing). Centres which elected radical surgery (mainly those in Germany and Austria), those which relied above all on radiation therapy, and those which proposed mixed approaches, had comparable long-term survival rates. International comparison also made it clear that even in the best cancer-treatment centres, which applied the most advanced therapeutic methods, the overall rates of cure of cervical malignancy were not very high. The main reason was the one indicated by Janet Lane-Claypon: many women were diagnosed with disseminated cervical malignancies. For example, gynaecologists from the Mayo Clinic (Rochester, MN, USA) found in the 1930s that 75% of their patients were diagnosed with stage III and IV tumours, and had therefore low chances of cure. Many specialists arrived at the conclusion that a perfection of the existing therapeutic methods might not be enough. The best way to reduce mortality from cervical cancer was to find a way to increase the proportion of women diagnosed before their tumour had spread beyond the cervix. The next important episode in the history of cervical cancer was the development of new diagnostic approaches.

4

THE PAP SMEAR

Looking for cervical lesions

In the early twentieth century, numerous cancer experts believed that if women could be persuaded to consult doctors immediately after they had noticed suspicious gynaecological symptoms, above all irregular bleeding, they would be diagnosed with stage I cancer (limited to the cervix) and would have an excellent chance of being cured. Alas, they realized that this was not the case. Many women who consulted their doctors quickly were still diagnosed with more advanced tumours (stages II and III), and many among them died from their disease. It was important to find a way to detect cervical tumours before any symptoms arose. In 1924 German gynaecologist Hans Hinselmann (1884–1959), from Hamburg, constructed an instrument destined to facilitate the search for suspicious changes in the cervix. This instrument, constructed in collaboration with the optical instrument company Leitz, was a specially adapted binocular microscope, fixed, mounted on a tripod, and equipped with a light source and a mirror to direct the light. Hinselmann named it the colposcope (from *col* meaning cervix and *scope* meaning looking at). Examination of the cervix through a colposcope, Hinselmann argued, made possible the detection of considerably earlier cancers. Even a tiny, dot-like tumour did not escape detection, but only if the observer was well trained, and had long experience of use of the colposcope. The need for a long period of training before becoming a competent colposcopist hampered the diffusion of Hinselmann's method, especially outside German-speaking countries.

Working with the colposcope, Hinselmann had found out that when he painted the cervix with dilute acetic acid zones of abnormal proliferation of cervical cells became visible as white patches. Such areas were then examined carefully with the colposcope, and often explored through biopsy. Around 1928, a Vienna gynaecologist, Walter Schiller (1887–1960), proposed to replace acetic acid with diluted iodine (Lugol stain). Normal cervical cells contain glycogen and absorb iodine, while rapidly proliferating abnormal cells do not store glycogen and remain white on a dark background. Gynaecologists who made biopsies of zones that remained white after staining with acetic acid or diluted iodine found in some cases an early cancer of the cervix. In other cases they found 'cancer-like' lesions. Cells in these lesions looked like cancer cells, but they remained on the surface of the cervix. Such superficial, cancer-like lesions lacked one of the main properties of cancer: the capacity to invade adjacent tissues.

Hinselmann and Schiller were not the first to observe superficial lesions of the cervix. The British gynaecologist John Williams (1840–1926) described such cancer-like lesions in 1888. Williams had found them when he examined a young woman with a gynaecological ailment. He believed that he had stumbled by chance on a very rare case. The results of biopsies of the white zones observed when the cervix was painted with acetic acid or Lugol stain indicated that superficial lesions of the cervix were not as rare as initially thought. Such 'precancerous' lesions of the cervix, many experts believed, played an important role in the development of malignant tumours. An Australian gynaecologist, Francis Matter, explained in 1935 that:

> the author is impressed and almost obsessed with the possibility of reducing cancer mortality in women by an early treatment and the discovery of the precancerous state. It is further suggested that health centers should advise women to be examined every year after the age of thirty. Great aid can be given to this examination by the use of Hinselmann's colposcope.[1]

Once such lesions were diagnosed, the next important question was what should be done about them. Walter Schiller was persuaded that non-invasive cervical lesions were an early stage of a true—that is, invasive—cancer. He determined all the intermediate stages between these two conditions. The demonstration of continuity between superficial lesions of the cervix and invasive cancer, was, Schiller argued, definitive proof that these lesions were indeed early stages of cervical cancer. Superficial lesions lacked some of the properties of a fully fledged cancer, but to deny the direct links between the two would be like denying that an embryo will become a newborn animal because the two do not look exactly the same. We do not speak of a 'pre-human embryo' but about a human one; similarly we should speak of an 'early cancer', not a 'precancerous condition'.[2] Schiller concluded that one should treat an 'early carcinoma of the cervix' exactly in the same way as an invasive cancer. A woman diagnosed with this condition should undergo a radical hysterectomy, and this operation would save her life.

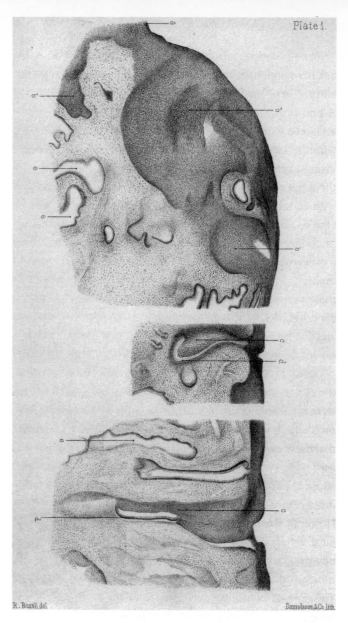

Plate 1.

R. Boxall, del.

Danielsson.&Co. lith.

2. Image of precancerous lesion of the cervix, by John Williams.
Wellcome Library, London.

Not all the specialists agreed with Schiller's view. Cancers, Schiller's opponents argued, have two properties: uncontrollable proliferation of cells and the capacity to invade other tissues. A 'non-invasive cancer' was a contradiction in terms. They also disagreed with the statement that all the white zones detected with the Lugol test were 'early cancers' which would become invasive tumours. The existence of intermediate states between the supposed early carcinoma and a late one did not establish with certainty that the second always evolved from the first. One could imagine simultaneous emergence of several kinds of abonormal cell arrangements, or even the possibility that a cancerous growth produced perturbations in the pattern of multiplication of cells in its vicinity. Moreover, even assuming that every invasive cancer developed from a non-invasive, cancer-like lesion, this did not mean that the opposite was true, and that every cancer-like lesion, or even an important proportion of these lesions, would became malignant.

Debates on the meaning of cancer-like superficial lesions of the cervix had important practical implications. Such lesions were often seen in young women who did not have any health problems. It was not clear whether doctors should recommend that these women undergo an ablation of the uterus, major surgery which might kill them and would make them sterile, or adopt a wait-and-see attitude, and put them at risk of a deadly disease. In the 1930s gynaecologists were divided on this issue. However, when some of the women diagnosed with a 'superficial carcinoma' of the cervix and left untreated developed invasive cancer, many gynaecologists concluded that it was more prudent to treat all women diagnosed with such a lesion. The only difference between the treatment of superficial and invasive cervical cancer was that in the first case doctors often performed a simple ablation of the uterus rather than the more extensive radical hysterectomy.

Catherine Macfarlane, a Philadelphia gynaecologist who started in 1938, together with another woman doctor, Margaret Sturgis, a pilot programme for the early detection of cervical cancer, made at that time an interesting proposal: to eliminate only suspicious cervical lesions. Every 6 months women enrolled in her programme underwent a careful visual inspection of the cervix. Invasive cancers (confirmed by biopsy) were treated with conventional means: surgery and/or radiation therapy. Superfical cervical lesions were simply eliminated: 'many conditions which might have led to cancer have been detected and corrected'.[3] Summing up the results of this preventive experiment in 1953, Catherine Macfarlane explained how she and her colleagues developed their innovative approach:

> at first we recommended quite a few biopsies. As we became more familiar with the appearance of a healthy cervix, our appreciation of the deviation therefore increased. We were less inclined to recommend spot biopsies and more inclined to recommend removal of the entire diseased area by circular biopsy or trachelectomy. By this means, the whole area was submitted to the pathologist, and a potentially cancerous lesion was removed at the same time.[4]

Catherine Mafarlane argued that when a women was diagnosed with a superficial cervical lesion the choice was not only between drastic surgery and inaction. It was possible to propose a third approach: the excision of the suspicious zones of the cervix. This was, Macfarlane believed, an efficient intervention. During the 15 years' duration of Macfarlane's pilot project, she and her collaborators found very few invasive cancers of the cervix. They attributed the relative rarity of malignant growths in their sample to the systematic surgical elimination of cervical lesions. In the 1940s and 1950s few cancer experts adopted this view. It became, however, increasingly popular from the 1960s onwards, following the widespread diffusion of a diagnostic technique which facilitated the identification of cervical lesions, the Pap smear.

Vaginal smears: the beginnings

In 1928 Dr George Papanicolaou (1893–1962), a pathologist of Greek origins who worked at the New York Hospital, wrote a short research paper in which he claimed that cervical smears could reveal hidden uterine cancers. Papanicolaou had a double training, in medicine and zoology. He worked for many years on the perfection of a laboratory test that measured the activity of oestrogen, a female sex hormone produced mainly by the ovaries. When administered to ovariectomized female mice this hormone was able to mimic the normal function of the ovary, and induce the female fertility cycle (oestrus). Papanicolaou found a simple way of measuring the appearance of oestrus: the observation of changes in cells in a vaginal smear. Mice injected with oestrogen preparations had typical changes in the vaginal lining, visible in vaginal smears. Papanicolaou's test became the standard way to measure oestrogen in commercial preparations. George Papanicolaou attempted then to apply the same method to 'human females' (his term) to study the biological activity of oestrogen in women. Such tests, he hoped, would facilitate the application of this hormone to treatment of disorders of the female cycle such as infertility or irregular menstruation. Papanicolaou realized then that he did not know what normal vaginal smears would look like. He examined smears from supposedly healthy women, and in some cases he saw unusual-looking cells. Gynaecological examination of these women showed that they had early cancer of the cervix. Papanicolaou had found accidentally a simple method to diagnose early cancer.

Papanicolaou's first publication on this subject described a small number of cases, and failed to persuade the experts. In 1941, Papanicolaou, together with a gynaecologist, Herbert Traut, published a more extended and more persuasive paper on the new method for the early detection of cervical malignancies:

> the present difficulty in accomplishing early diagnosis lies in the fact that we must depend on subjective symptoms of the disease to bring the patient to the physician, and by the time the patient becomes sufficiently aware of discomfort to seek help, the disease is far advanced....if by any chance a simple, inexpensive method of diagnosis could be evolved which could be applied to large numbers of women in the cancer-bearing period of life, we would be in a position to discover the disease in its incipiency much more frequently than is now possible.[5]

Papanicolaou's claims were confirmed by other researchers. A technical improvement, the introduction of a wooden spatula, facilitated the collection of cervical cells, and helped to make smears more reliable. Some gynaecologists quickly adopted this method—rapidly renamed the Papanicolaou or Pap smear—and systematically tested all the women in their practice. In the late 1940s some gynaecologists advocated the generalization of systematic screening using the Pap smear to all the women at risk of cervical cancer. At that stage, the goal of this test was to find early stages of invasive cancers, then to treat women diagnosed with early-stage malignant tumours with hysterectomy and/or radiation therapy. Women described in the original publication of Papanicolaou and Traut were either healthy or had a cancer. However, with extended use of the Pap smear gynaecologists saw a rapid increase in diagnoses of non-invasive, cancer-like lesions.

Treatment of superficial cancer of the cervix in the Pap-smear era

When a cervical smear was normal, or showed the presence of cancer cells, gynaecologists knew what they should do. When the smear was 'intermediary' or 'borderline'—not a rare event—they wished to pursue their investigations to learn more about the condition of the cervix. From the mid 1950s onwards gynae-cologists in North America and Western Europe increasingly employed Hinselmann's colposcope to examine women with doubtful results from the Pap smear. Many of these women underwent biopsies and some were diagnosed with superficial cancer-like lesions of the cervix, renamed carcinoma *in situ*. In the interwar era a superficial carcinoma of the cervix was occasionally found in women who went to see a gynaecologist because they had bothersome symptoms, but also in those per-suaded to undergo regular gynaecological check-ups to reduce their risk of developing cancer. At that time only a tiny fraction of women underwent such regular check-ups. By consequence the number of women diagnosed with superficial lesions of the cervix was not very large. However, use of the Pap smear led to a rapid increase in the number of diagnoses of cancer-like cervi-cal lesions. Dilemmas concerning the treatment of these lesions remained the same as in the interwar era, but in the 1950s and 1960s such dilemmas became much more frequent.

Specialists continued to be divided on the question of how dangerous carcinoma *in situ* of the cervix was. Seventy US gynae-cologists were asked in 1952 whether they believed in sponta-neous regression of cervical cancer *in situ*. Fourteen answered yes, 34 no, and 22 that they did not know.[6] Epidemiological data from the 1950s did not support Walter Schiller's hypothesis that all *in situ* cancers became invasive if left alone. Epidemiologists had found out that many more US women were diagnosed with non-invasive cervical lesions than with cervical cancer. They concluded that probably only between 10 and 15% of women diagnosed with *in situ* cancer would develop an invasive tumour.[7] One chance out of 7, or even 1 out of 10, of developing a deadly disease, was nevertheless a serious risk. In the 1950s, many gynaecologists continued therefore to adhere to the view that one is better safe than sorry, and treated women diagnosed with *in situ* carcinoma of the cervix with ablation of the uterus or radiation therapy. Only in exceptional cases did doctors try to conserve the fertility of a young woman and propose a par-tial ablation of the cervix instead of a complete hysterectomy.

The problem was further complicated by disagreement among the experts on the definition of carcinoma *in situ*. Pathologists proposed different definitions of mild, moderate, and severe dysplasia (a less severe lesion), and readily acknow-ledged that, one expert's dysplasia may be another's carcinoma *in situ*. For example, in 1956 25 US pathologists were sent 20 iden-tical 'borderline' slides, and were asked to determine how many among these preparations were from precancerous lesions and how many were from 'true' cancers. Three pathologists found no cancer, three a single case of malignancy, and, on the other end, four pathologists had found 9 cases of true cancer, one 12 cases, and one 13 such cases.[8]

Two studies made in the 1950s and 1960s led to important changes in the treatment of *in situ* carcinoma of the cervix. In a study made in Denmark by the gynaecologist Olaf Petersen some women diagnosed with *in situ* carcinoma of the cervix were treated with radiation therapy or hysterectomy, whereas other women had regular gynaecological examinations only (watchful waiting) for 10–15 years. There were no cancers among the treated women, but some women suffered from severe side effects of their therapy. Several of those in the watchful waiting group developed cervical cancers, nearly all of which were treated successfully. The majority of the women in the non-treated group remained, however, cancer-free, an observation that confirmed epidemiologists' conclusions that only a fraction of women with an *in situ* cancer develop invasive malignancies. Petersen concluded that cervical lesions usually evolve very slowly, and a diagnosis of a superficial carcinoma of the cervix is not a medical emergency. It was possible to propose to women diagnosed with such lesions to wait for some time and see how they would evolve. Petersen added, however, that this was not an absolute rule. In some cases, cervical lesions which looked relatively mild would change suddenly and unpredictably become more dangerous.[9]

Petersen and his colleagues believed that dangerous-looking lesions should be treated through hysterectomy or radiation therapy. In the 1960s US gynaecologists found that superficial cervical lesions are very fragile. This observation was an unexpected result of a study that aimed at a better understanding of the natural history of cervical dysplasia (an abnormal proliferation of cells, a term that includes *in situ* carcinoma and other cancer-like lesions). The US gynaecologist Leopold Koss and his collaborators selected women with cervical dysplasia, made a biopsy of their cervical lesion, then asked them to come back several months later for a second biopsy to be made of the same lesion. To their surprise, at the second visit they were unable to find the lesions that they studied during the first visit. Biopsy was sufficient to destroy these lesions, and therefore to cure them. Dysplasia and carcinoma *in situ* of the cervix, Koss and his colleagues concluded, are often extremely fragile structures, and can be eliminated easily through minor surgery. Their study failed to achieve its goal, but it had accidentally stumbled on a simple way to eliminate cervical lesions.[10] Catherine Macfarlane was right. It was possible to prevent cervical cancer, and a biopsy could be a curative, and not only a diagnostic approach.

In the late 1960s cervical cancer entered an era of preventive medicine. In the 1970s gynaecologists developed a surgical procedure, called conic biopsy, destined to eliminate cervical lesions. They also elaborated alternative methods for the destruction of these lesions: thermocoagulation (killing with heat), cryotherapy (killing by low temperatures), and laser treatment. Specialists had found out that such local interventions worked well in 90% of the cases. In the remaining 10% the procedure could be repeated a few months later. Only in a small number of resistant cases did it become necessary to perform more extended surgery, usually ablation of the cervix, and in some cases the whole uterus. The finding that a simple local treatment eliminated the danger of cervical cancer radically changed the goals of screening for *in situ* lesions of the cervix. Originally such screening was expected to uncover an early aggressive cancer, then to get rid of it with an equally aggressive treatment. Later, however, the aim of screening was redefined as the elimination of a weak, poorly established precancerous lesion with conservative surgical methods.

The finding that it is relatively easy to destroy cervical lesions lessened the pressure for an accurate diagnosis of such lesions. Pathologists still disagreed whether a given lesion should be classified as moderate or severe dysplasia, and continued to propose somewhat discordant definitions of carcinoma *in situ*. However, once they adopted the principle that every suspicious cervical lesion should be removed, the only important distinction became the one between lesions that may be left alone and those that need to be treated:

> If one accepts that cervical intraepithelial neoplasia (*in situ* lesions) is a continuous process, then the grade of de-differentiation is principally a statement of probability of development of an invasive carcinoma, but such an aggregate probability statement is meaningless for the individual patient. The important element for a woman diagnosed with a proliferative lesion of the cervix is the ease of elimination of a suspicious lesion and not details of its histological diagnosis. Hence, the important diagnostic categories are: normal cervix, cervical intraepithelial neoplasia, microinvasion and invasive carcinoma. Thanks to generalization of colposcopy and a greater experience of clinicians to recognize abnormal histology, 95% of cases are treated locally.[11]

The switch to less aggressive treatment of superficial lesions of the cervix was gradual, but in the 1980s harsh therapies for such lesions were near universally replaced with relatively simple treatments that could often be performed under local anaesthesia. On the other hand, when treatment of cervical lesions was reclassified as minor surgery doctors were more often inclined to propose such a treatment to all the women who faced a risk of cervical cancer, however slight. Many women, who in all probability would never have developed an invasive cancer, underwent a minor but not inconsequential treatment which sometimes produced temporary problems (pain, uncontrolled bleeding), and, in rare cases, more severe complications (such as sterility). The question of the threshold of intervention—the decision when doctors had the obligation to act for their patient, and when the best choice was to refrain from intervention— was at the centre of a highly publicized 'scandal' of treatment of women with an *in situ* cancer of the cervix at New Zealand's National Women's Hospital.

The 'scandal' at the New Zealand National Women's Hospital

In June 1987 Sandra Coney, journalist and feminist activist, and Phillida Bunkle, senior lecturer in Women's Studies at Victoria University, Wellington, New Zealand, published in Auckland's *Metro* magazine a text that strongly criticized the inadequate treatment of women with cervical lesions at New Zealand National Women's Hospital. The scandal at the Women's Hospital became a *cause célèbre* in New Zealand. It was presented as an example of callous and insensitive treatment of women by male doctors, and illegitimate medical experimentation. The story of this scandal started in the 1950s, when one of the leading gynaecologists of the New Zealand Women's Hospital, Herbert Green (1916–2001), concerned by what he saw as an excessive surgical activism by gynaecologists, proposed more conservative treatment of women diagnosed with *in situ* cancer of the cervix. A few among Green's patients developed invasive cancers. Green's approach was probably akin to the study conducted by Olaf Petersen in Copenhagen in the 1940s and 1950s. The main difference was that Petersen explicitly presented his study as a clinical trial, although it is not clear whether his patients knew that they took part in such a trial. Green, unlike Petersen, did not see himself as conducting a clinical experiment. He believed that he treated all his patients according to what he saw as the best available standards of care, and decided in each case what would be the most appropriate way to deal with his patients' *in situ* cancer.

Some of Green's colleagues at the New Zealand's Women's Hospital disagreed with his views. In 1984 the hospital's cytologist and pathologist published an article in an American medical journal in which they argued that patients diagnosed with carcinoma *in situ* at the National Women's Hospital, and who continued to have positive Pap smears 2 years after their initial diagnosis, were 12 times more likely to develop an invasive cancer than women who were treated and had reverted to a negative smear. *In situ* cervical lesions, they argued, should be eliminated at all costs. Their article was an open critique of Green's therapeutic approach. At first the debate on the best way to treat women with *in situ* carcinoma of the cervix was conducted among specialists. Sandra Coney's and Phillida Bunkle's 1987 article brought it to the attention of the general public. Herbert Green, their article claimed, had allowed women to develop cervical cancer as part of a medical experiment on conservative treatment of this lesion. Coney and Bunkle's interpretation was later accepted by a Committee of Inquiry appointed by the New Zealand government (the Cartwright Cancer Commission), which strongly criticized Green's therapeutic approach.

Green's accusers—supported by some of his colleagues at the hospital—pointed to the problematic outcomes of his approach for some women, and to the fact that these women were not informed about the existence of alternative therapeutic approaches. Some of the women who later developed cancer accused Green of unethical behaviour, and some journalists and activists transformed Green into a symbol of the unfeeling, arrogant male doctor who manipulated and harmed women's bodies. The medical historian Linda Bryder believes that such a view of Green's treatment of women with *in situ* cancer of the cervix, was not only excessive, but totally false. Bryder, who published in 2009 a careful and well-documented study of the accusations against Green and their background, argues there was no consensus about the treatment of cervical carcinoma *in situ*. When Green promoted a conservative therapy of this lesion (which included conic biopsies, when appropriate) he did not conduct an illegitimate experiment on sick women but exploited one of the legitimate options available at that time. Other gynaecologists proposed a similar approach to treatment of *in situ* cancer of the cervix (although, one may add, in the 1960s this was not a majority point of view). Moreover, Bryder explains, the whole notion of 'experiment' developed by the report of the Cartwright Commission was artificially constructed from partial and inaccurate data.[12] Bryder's book reopened a debate on the 'scandal' at the New Zealand National Women's Hospital. A collective book, with contributions by some of the original contributors to the Cartwright Cancer Committee inquiry, and by other scholars, sustains that the commission's conclusions were correct and that Green's behaviour was indeed unethical.[13] The fact that 30 years after Green's retirement his treatment of cervical carcinoma *in situ* still produces passionate debates is an apt illustration of the controversial nature of this topic.

The Latin American exception: the use of colposcope for screening for cervical lesions

From the 1940s onwards Western countries adopted the use of vaginal smears to look for cervical cancer and premalignant lesions of the cervix. Some Latin American countries, above all Argentina and Brazil, elected a different path: the perfection of the 'pre Pap smear' pattern of screening grounded in a direct examination of the cervix, usually with Hinselmann's colposcope. The history of detection of cervical lesions in South America was partly the result of the unbroken influence of the German–Austrian school of gynaecology in Latin America. The arrival of the Nazis to power in Germany, then the Second World War, interrupted the professional relationships between gynaecologists in North America and Western Europe and those in German-speaking countries. By contrast, Argentinian and Brazilian gynaecologists, many of whom were trained in Germany or Austria, maintained close contacts with colleagues in these countries. Such uninterrupted German influence favoured the adoption of colposcopy for the search for cervical cancer and premalignant lesions.

Colposcopy was introduced into Argentina by Dr Alfredo Jakob. Jakob trained with Hinselmann in Hamburg in 1932. He returned to Argentina in 1933, and brought this technique to the Maternity Hospital in Buenos Aires. He also offered training courses in this technique for his colleagues. Many Buenos Aires gynaecologists adopted colposcopy as a reliable method of early detection of cervical cancer. The supporters of this technique saw it as superior to vaginal smears because it made possible direct observation of the cervix and the immediate evaluation of the potential danger of cervical lesions. They also believed that it was possible to extend the use of this technique to screen all healthy women.

The diffusion of colposcopy in Argentina was further promoted by the frequent travels of Hinselmann to South America. After the war Hinselmann was condemned for illegal 'racial' sterilization of gypsy women. His name was also linked, without formal proof, with experiments on prisoners conducted in Auschwitz by his ex-student and close collaborator, Eduard Wirths. Hinselmann spent 3 years in prison and was stripped of his academic privileges. He saw himself as a victim of injustice, arguing that the sterilization of gypsy women was conducted in the framework of the Nazi race hygiene laws, and was therefore perfectly legal. When he regained his freedom, Hinselmann, who lost much of his professional standing in Germany, was delighted to find intact the friendship, support, and admiration of his Latin American followers. He described his enthusiastic reception in Brazil and Argentina as 'a corner of a blue sky'.

In 1951 Hinselmann was invited by Dr Ahumada, the head of the gynaecology clinic at Buenos Aires National University, to teach colposcopy to medical students. He extended his visit for 4 months, during which he gave many conferences, travelled tirelessly to the hospitals of Brazil, Argentina, and Uruguay, and organized numerous training courses on colposcopy. By the 1950s the main gynaecological clinics in Buenos Aires, and in some cities of Argentina's interior, had opened colposcopy departments. Many gynaecologists across the country referred patients to centres that possessed the instruments to examine their suspected cervical lesions.

Colposcopy was introduced to Brazil by Armando de Moraes (1893–1961), professor of gynaecology at the Medical School of Brazil University, Rio de Janeiro. De Moraes's student, Joao Paulo

Rieper, studied with Hans Hinselmann in Hamburg, and in 1942 published a thesis on the practical value of colposcopy. De Moraes was also interested in cervical smears. As early as 1942 (thus 1 year after the publication of Papanicolaou and Traut's article on this technique) another of his students wrote a thesis on the use of Pap smears for the detection of cervical tumours. The publication in the same year of two MD theses on two different methods to detect cervical lesions was not due to chance. Armando de Moraes advocated the combined use of these two techniques for an early diagnosis of cervical malignancies. He and his students elaborated a unique 'triple model' of detection of cervical lesions, which combined colposcopy, cytology, and histopathology. Women underwent at the same time a gynaecological examination with a colposcope, a cervical smear, and, if necessary, a cervical biopsy. The triple method, its advocates claimed, provided the best chance to detect cervical anomalies. It was a labour-intensive approach, but on the other hand an immediate and accurate diagnosis reduced the costs of additional tests and repeated visits to the clinics. It also limited the number of false-negative results and unnecessary treatments.

In 1948 the Gynaecological Institute in Rio de Janeiro, directed by Armando de Moraes, opened a Preventive Dispensary of Gynaecological Cancer. The name 'preventive', the founders of this dispensary recognized later, was chosen mainly for psychological reasons. The original aim of the dispensary was to detect already existing cancers, but 'prevention' sounded less ominous. Later, however, the Rio dispensary did became a centre for prevention of cancer, since one of its main goals became diagnosis and elimination of precancerous lesions. The dispensary adopted the triple model. João Paulo Rieper was responsible for colposcopic examinations, Clarice do Amaral Ferreira, a gynaecologist trained in cytology, took over the reading of Pap smears, and another woman physician, Hildegard Stoltz, organized the data on diagnosis and treatments. The main task of this dispensary was didactical: a demonstration of the feasibility of the triple model and the promotion of this approach in Brazil. Armando de Moraes and his colleagues were successful. In the 1950s and 1960s colposcopy was integrated by many Brazilian gynaecologists into the routine examination of their patients. These specialists inverted the order of search methods for cervical lesions. In Western countries the rule was to do a Pap smear first, and only if a cervical smear detected abnormal cells would the physician send the patient for a colposcopic examination. In Argentina and Brazil many gynaecologists first examined the cervix through the colposcope and then, if they found suspicious changes, prepared a cervical smear and sent it to the cytology laboratory. Both approaches can be presented as logical, but only the former became a routine method for detection of cervical lesions.

Looking for cervical lesions in the twenty-first century: persisting uncertainties

One of the most problematic aspects of screening for cervical cancer is the difficulty of finding out what the exact meaning of a positive result is. Three parallel systems of classification of cervical lesions co-exist today. The system promoted by the World Health Organization (WHO) and the Pan-American Health Organization (PAHO) distinguishes between mild, moderate, and severe dysplasia (abnormal proliferation of cells) and then carcinoma *in situ*. The Richart system, used mainly by colposcopists, differentiates three stages of cervical intraepithelial neoplasia (a collective name for cervical lesions): CIN-1, CIN-2, and CIN-3. Finally the Bethesda classification, often employed by cytopathologists and cytotechnicians, differentiates between low-grade squamous intraepithelial lesion (LSIL) and high-grade squamous intraepithelial lesion (HSIL). Mild dysplasia corresponds to CIN-1 and LSIL; moderate dysplasia to CIN-2 and part of the HSIL spectrum; severe dysplasia and carcinoma *in situ* are lumped together in the CIN-3 definition, and, together with moderate dysplasia, are part of the HSIL spectrum. The correspondence between these three systems is, however, imperfect, and the definition of borderline cases within each system depends partly on the idiosyncratic preferences of individual pathologists.

All the classifications maintain a certain level of ambiguity. Isolated cells from a cervical smear, scraped from the cervix with a wooden spatula and put on a microscopic slide, are often classified using terms which usually refer to the organization of tissues, such as 'lesion' (in LSIL and HSIL) and 'neoplasia' (in CIN). The implicit assumption is that the results of Pap smears faithfully mirror the presence of well-defined pathological changes in the cervix. This is far, however, from being the case. A non-negligible percentage of screened women (on average 1 in 15 to 1 in 20 women who undergo a Pap smear) receive a diagnosis of atypical squamous cells of unknown significance (ASCUS). In plain language, this term means that doctors do not know what the meaning of the observed changes in cells scraped from the cervix is. When the diagnosis is uncertain, follow-up recommendations are uncertain too. Many gynaecologists see an ACSUS diagnosis as indicating the need for more frequent cervical smears. The great majority of lesions that produce ASCUS, they argue, are slow-growing, or regress spontaneously, justifying a wait-and-see attitude. Other specialists point to the fact that 5–10% of women with ASCUS have more dangerous (high-grade) lesions, and a few may even have an invasive cancer. They recommend therefore a colposcopy, and a biopsy. The latter tests may, however, also end by being inconclusive.[14] Many women find themselves in a diagnostic 'no man's land'. They hover between health and disease, and wonder whether their womb, previously seen as an unproblematic part of their body, harbours a ticking bomb.

An efficient but not entirely benign procedure

Jade Goody received several warnings about abnormal Pap smears and failed to act upon these warnings. Her behaviour may be dismissed as irresponsible. It may also be an indication of a real and rarely discussed problem: the elimination of cervical lesions is sometimes a traumatic event for the patient. Goody affirmed that the treatment she underwent at the age of 16 was so painful that she dreaded the repetition of this experience. It is not excluded that, in her case, the pain was amplified by her apprehension of cancer, lack of understanding of what was happening in her body, and absence of an accurate and honest explanation of what she should expect during and after her treatment.

Many women are reluctant to undergo gynaecological examination with a speculum, not only because they find this examination embarrassing, but also because the insertion of a speculum, especially by an inexperienced or careless physician, may be uncomfortable and sometimes painful. Even in the twenty-first century, many women dislike repeated gynaecological examinations, and, as the US journalist Lisa Spinelli put it, 'being poked like a stuffed pig'. This is even more true for biopsies: the slicing of small bits of tissue. This procedure may be quite painful, even if it is done under local anaesthesia, which is far from being a rule. Spinelli described her cervical biopsy, made after two positive Pap smears:

> a not-exactly-awesome procedure called the endocervical curettage that involves a doctor scraping the canal between the cervix and the uterus with a thing that looks like a long metal file. Sound like a party? Cramp-like symptoms, check; bleeding, check; exhaustion, check.[15]

Gynaecologists, cancer experts, and cancer organizations who advocate the systematic supervision of women's bodies for early signs of cervical cancer discuss the need to overcome women's false modesty and shame, but seldom mention the discomfort of the preparation of cervical smears, and the fact that a positive smear may lead to more distressing diagnostic tests. There are few discussions on unpleasantness linked with screening for cervical cancer in the professional literature, and the topic is practically invisible in public debates on screening, perhaps because the absence of an organized movement of women with cervical cancer. In this regard, cervical cancer is very different from breast cancer, a disease made highly visible in the last 30 years, mainly thanks to the rise of a strong patient movement. Organizations which loudly voice concerns about breast cancer and offer women spaces to discuss their experience with this disease came into being in the aftermath of AIDS epidemics, and were modelled on AIDS activism, developed in the 1980s. At that time, cervical cancer was no longer seen as an important health problem in Western countries.

Another possible reason for the lack of debate on the unpleasant consequences of diagnosis of suspected cervical lesions is

the doctor's difficulty in acknowledging the pain and discomfort produced by routine diagnostic procedures. Physicians
and other health professionals tend to overlook the fact that
interventions which they define as 'minor' are not necessarily seen as minor by their patients. An Israeli journalist, Vered
Levi-Barzilai, described the extreme pain she suffered during a
biopsy of the endometrium, which is a test done, among other
things, to detect the presence of cancer of the uterine body. She
was told that the procedure is simple and rapid and produces
only slight discomfort, then found herself suffering intense pain
that made her cry out. She asked later why she was not given
anaesthesia and was told that, 'apparently, you have an unusual
pain threshold'. 'It's not a procedure that justifies sedation', said
one gynaecologist who was asked for his opinion. 'Maybe you
were a little hysterical going into the test? Stress adds to pain, it's
a known thing', he added. 'You must be exaggerating. It couldn't
have hurt you that much', asserted another senior gynaecologist. A short enquiry among her friends uncovered that all those
who underwent this test without anaesthesia had the same
opinion:

> all the stories were nearly identical: it was a nightmare. The
> doctor said it wouldn't hurt; it was done in a regular gynae-
> cologist's office without any sort of anaesthetic. Why? Just
> because. That's the protocol.[16]

'The something of nothing': women's experience of screening for cervical cancer

One of the arguments advanced by advocates of regular screening for cervical cancer is that the great majority of women
receive a negative result (there are no abnormal cells in the

smear) and are reassured that they are fine. This is true for some, but not for all women. An invitation to be tested may be a remainder of the possibility of cancer. An Australian woman tried to make sense of the meaning of cervical cancer, a disease she even did not think about before her Pap smear:

> so I thought, now I'll look this up in a medical book. But that wasn't so good, I looked up cervical cancer and then I discovered 'my gosh, people die!' And then I don't know if it said this exactly, but as I remember, so, if you discover it early, then 85 per cent make it. And I don't know anything, I'm not a doctor or anything, so I interpreted it like, 'oy, 15 per cent die', that's one-and-a-half people out of 10 that die when you discover it early. And then I really ... went into a depression or had death anxiety.[17]

Moreover, a non-negligible percentage of women receive an unclear result of a Pap smear. Such results may destabilize their view of themselves as healthy, and undermine their confidence in their bodies. A doctor's reassurance that a mild anomaly is 'just nothing', may be interpreted in an opposite way, as an indication that there is something deeply wrong in the woman's body. Another Australian woman testified that:

> they told me that this was nothing to worry about, and it wasn't so dangerous and that I would come and have a test ... in any case, I said that I wasn't going to wait ... you get scared, in any case, I got scared ... got the feeling that, yes, what can this turn into? ... The doctor told me that mild dysplasia is really nothing except that the degree of change is small. Then if it's cancer or not, she said, that has to be shown in the next test.[18]

Positive results from a Pap smear may produce a different type of problem. Jade Goody described her preventive treatment as highly distressing. The medical sociologist, Nicky Britten, who, unlike Jade Goody, has a good understanding of the reasons for screening for cervical malignancies, and a decidedly positive attitude towards such a screening, also described her treatment of cervical dysplasia as a traumatic event. When Britten learned about the presence of abnormal cells in her cervical smear, for several days she was unable to think about anything but death. She was also shaken by the side effects of her treatment such as pain and uncontrolled bleeding, the more so because nobody informed her about the possibility of these complications. The experience, Britten explained:

> has not left me unchanged. Is it as if, having allowed the possibility of one disease to enter my body, a host of other conditions have crowded behind it.... I lost an innocence of outlook.[19]

Scholars who are fully persuaded that screening for cervical tumours is a good thing still believe that it is important to give adequate information on the hazards of screening for one's mental and physical health to allow the woman to make truly informed choices. Tests such as the Pap smear are neither neutral nor anodyne, and it is not unreasonable to ask that they should be submitted to the same rules on informed consent as other medical interventions.

Another negative effect of screening may be the false certitude that 'doing everything right' and having regular Pap smears will provide absolute protection from cervical cancer. The US science journalist Shanon Brownlee told the story of a woman who was treated for abnormal cervical cells and believed to be cured, because the following Pap smears were negative. Alas, in spite of the negative tests, she developed an incurable cervical malignancy. Learning about her cancer, she became furious, and remained so until her death:

> she was so angry because she has done everything right in her mind. She went to the doctor like a clockwork, she never missed an appointment for her Pap. She thought, if I do what I'm supposed to do, I will get my gold star from heaven; I will be protected. Then God violated the contract. It was bad enough that she died at age of forty, but she was so angry, she would not even say goodbye to her children.[20]

The observation that screening for cervical cancer can occasionally produce harm is usually interpreted as a call for greater prudence, not as contestation of the value of such screening. The majority of gynaecologists, public health experts, and activists strongly support the generalization of Pap smears. Early detection of some malignant tumours, such as prostate or lung cancers, is controversial. This is not the case in the search for cervical lesions. The widespread agreement on the desirability of such a search led to efforts to extend this screening to all the women at risk of this disease. From the early twentieth century on, cancer experts and cancer charities energetically advocated early detection of uterine cancer. The subsequent development of an efficient method of observation of precancerous lesions of the cervix and of elimination of these lesions led to the definition of cervical cancer as a public health problem and the development of large-scale screening campaigns.

5

SAVE THE WOMEN

The early roots of a public health policy

The early diagnosis of cancer is of interest only if one assumes that cancer starts as a local disorder, and is curable at that stage. Doctors who were persuaded that cancer of the uterus was a hereditary, incurable disease did not have any reason to encourage women who noticed symptoms such as an irregular bleeding to consult them rapidly. They were not in a hurry to deliver bad news. By contrast, those who believed that cancer of the womb always starts as a local 'sore', which could be treated, wanted their patients to visit them as rapidly as possible. Cancer of the womb, the French physician Julien Bertre complained in 1824, is a very frustrating disease for the doctor, because he or she is usually called only when the sole treatment that can be proposed is a generous dose of painkillers. The main problem, Bertre added, was women's reluctance to see a doctor when their disease was at an early, curable stage: 'because of praiseworthy modesty, they consult too late'.[1] Calls for the early detection of uterine tumours were less frequent in the mid nineteenth century, when many physicians lost faith in the possibility of curing this ailment. Renewed faith in surgical solutions in the late nineteenth century led to a return of interest in the early detection of cancer of the uterus, then to efforts to systematically promote such detection through education of professionals and the lay public.

In the early twentieth century, physicians in several countries—Austria, Germany, Hungary, Switzerland, and the USA—made systematic efforts to teach women, doctors, midwives, and nurses about early signs of cancer of the uterus. Women who came to gynaecological clinics in Austria and Hungary were handed leaflets explaining that if they suffered from irregular vaginal bleeding they needed to see a doctor immediately. At the same time, general practitioners (GPs), midwives, nurses, and pharmacists received more detailed information about early signs of cancer of the uterus and the importance of rapid surgical intervention. The most-quoted early example of the successful diffusion of information about uterine tumours was the campaign conducted by Dr Winter at Königsberg, formerly in East Prussia, now in Germany. Winter claimed that, thanks to this campaign, the percentage of women diagnosed with an 'operable' cancer of the uterus increased from 21 to 74%.[2]

The British surgeon Charles Childe, a pioneer of cancer education in the UK, believed that educators—above all health professionals who were in direct contact with patients—should fight two erroneous perceptions: the exclusive linking of cancer with pain and loss of weight, and the view that cancer cannot be cured, or, alternatively, that the cure is worse than the disease. A leaflet published in 1906 by the Gynaecological and Obstetrical Society of Roman Switzerland, and written for lay people, warned women against prevarication when they observed suspicious symptoms such as irregular vaginal bleeding, or bleeding after menopause: 'we do not wish to scare you without a reason, but when we observe this negligence, this loss of time, that so often led to loss of life of mothers, it is our duty to raise an energetic alarm cry'.[3]

Campaigns in favour of the early detection of cervical cancer before the Pap smear

In the interwar era cancer organizations conducted educational campaigns about the early signs of cancer. These campaigns focused, as a rule, on female tumours of the breast and uterus. In the 1920s and 1930s cancer was still seen as a women's disease. Moreover, cancers of the breast and uterus, the main causes of cancer mortality among women, produced typical symptoms (a lump in the breast, irregular bleeding) before they reached an incurable stage. By contrast, cancer often found in men— stomach, gut, liver, or lung—was often manifested only when it was too late to attempt a cure. The conviction that cancer education should be targeted above all at women was summed up in a US 1939 poster that boldly stated 'More women die of cancer than do men. 70 percent of the 35,000 women who die annually from cancer of the breast and uterus could be saved if treated in time'.[4]

In the 1930s, documents of the main British cancer organization, the British Empire Cancer Campaign (BECC), authoritatively affirmed that between 80 and 90% of patients diagnosed with early-stage breast or uterine cancer were alive 5 years after their treatment, as compared with a 20–30% 5-year survival rate for patients diagnosed with later stages of the disease. The implicit message was that prompt consultation of doctors would transform these cancers into curable diseases. BECC members who gave public talks were instructed to focus on breast and uterine cancer, especially if the audience was female: 'by contrast, it is a poor idea to speak about stomach cancer. There is no early diagnosis, and people with slight indigestion will believe they have cancer.'[5] The French *Ligue contre le Cancer* and the American Society for the Control of Cancer (ASCC) also focused their educational activities on female cancers.

Joseph Colt Bloodgood (1867–1935), Johns Hopkins surgeon and one of the most important cancer experts in the USA in the early twentieth century, became an indefatigable promoter of the early detection of uterine tumours. In an article published in 1927 in the popular US women's magazine *Good Housekeeping* he explained that 'false modesty, chiefly on the part of the public press, has make it difficult to get the correct information to the public'.[6] In 1930 Bloodgood founded the Amanda Sims Memorial Fund (ASMF), named after the wife of the donor who helped to establish the fund, the carpenter John E. Sims. The goal of ASMF was to raise women's awareness about cancer of the womb. ASMF activists spread the message about the need to pay attention to gynaecological symptoms among women's organizations and women's clubs. ASMF was one of the sources of inspiration of the ASCC's Women's Field Army, founded in the 1930s to disseminate educational messages about female cancers, especially through networks of women's clubs. Field Army activists repeated the injunction that women who noticed suspicious gynaecological manifestations, however insignificant, should see their doctors as soon as possible.

In the 1930s doctors increasingly realized, however, that cancer of the cervix did not always produce early warning signs. Many women who consulted immediately when they noticed unusual symptoms had already missed a good chance of cure. US pioneer of screening for cervical tumours, Catherine Macfarlane, explained that,

> an attempt was made to acquaint the women of Philadelphia with the signs and symptoms of pelvic cancer and to convince them of the need for consulting a physician as soon as such symptoms appeared. From time to time, as a result of this campaign, women would present themselves a few days or a few weeks after their first symptom, and yet examination will reveal a pelvic cancer in an advanced stage. These cases led us to conclude that the best way to detect pelvic cancer in an early and curable stage might be by the periodic pelvic examination of presumably well women.[7]

Other specialists agreed. The bulletin of the French *Ligue contre le Cancer* reported in 1928 that the New York chapter of the ASCC had opened 'cancer clinics' which, among other things, provided gynaecological check-ups for healthy women. The upper part of the body of a woman who underwent such a check-up, the French visitor noticed with admiration, was hidden behind a screen, providing 'a perfectly anonymous examination'.[8] French cancer experts such as Claudius Regaud and Simone Laborde advocated in the early 1930s periodic gynaecological examinations for all women (besides the very young and the very old). Such preventive medical visits (by that time French experts already called them screening consultations) should be paid for through the patient's health insurance. Claudius Regaud proposed in 1932 that when the Curie Foundation opened a new hospital dedicated to the treatment of cancer it would include a dispensary specializing in such early detection of cervical malignancies.[9] Simone Laborde even considered the possibility of introducing obligatory or semi-obligatory gynaecological check-ups, because with persuasion alone 'we will be obliged to wait many years before the generalization of this practice'.[10]

Walter Schiller proposed in 1933 to use his Lugol test (the painting of the cervix with dilute iodine) to promote the detection of localized cervical lesions:

> if every woman would have twice or three times a year a routine Lugol test, it would be possible to locate a carcinoma of the cervix in its earlier stages and treatment could immediately be instituted that would raise the percentage of complete healing to 95 or 100%...such a routine examination would not involve great expense, and would not require especially instructed men.[11]

He reiterated this proposal 5 years later. At that time he came to the conclusion that cervical cancer usually develops slowly and has a long period of surface growth before it starts to invade other tissues. For this reason, a regular search for early tumours of the cervix is an especially efficient way to reduce mortality from this malignancy. In January 1937 Schiller presented this idea at the annual meeting of the American Society for the Advancement of Science. *Time* magazine reported that:

> Dr Walter Schiller of the University of Vienna offered a simple new way of determining whether or not a woman has cancer of the cervix. He paints it with iodine. If the cervix is healthy, the iodine makes the surface turn blue. If there is the slightest trace of cancer, the spot will turn white. Dr. Schiller urged all women to have the iodine test every six months, or at least once a year.[12]

Walter Schiller observed cervical lesions with the colposcope. At that time, however, very few US gynaecologists were familiar with the use of this instrument (in the 1930s, the colposcope was employed mainly in German-speaking countries), and even fewer were trained to recognize early cervical lesions. An additional obstacle to the organization of an effective mass-screening campaign for cervical cancer might have been the fact that the disease was especially frequent among poor women, who could not afford to see a gynaecologist.

The last point may be illustrated by the failure of the first campaign for the early detection of cervical tumours organized by Catherine Macfarlane in Philadelphia in the USA. Macfarlane was aware of the high occurrence of cervical cancer among poor women in the city. Many of these women were of African American origin. She had learned that campaigns to screen women for cervical cancer with pelvic examinations and colposcopy worked well in East Prussia, and in the 1930s she decided to conduct a similar campaign in Philadelphia. Her original choice to rely only on a simple visual inspection of the cervix was linked to an aspiration to provide inexpensive services to women from lower social strata. Macfarlane's initiative was, however, opposed by the local medical community and by the administrators of the Women's Medical College to which she was affiliated. Doctors feared interference with their private practice and some suspected that the programme proposed by Macfarlane had left-wing connotations.

The Women's Medical College finally approved Macfarlane's project, but made her agree to limit it to the screening of women referred to her by their own physicians. This restriction aimed to overcome doctors' fears that they would lose their private patients to Macfarlane's and similar programmes. This condition efficiently destroyed Catherine Macfarlane's original goal. Cervical cancer rates were much lower among affluent women who could afford regular visits to a private practitioner than among the disadvantaged population originally targeted by

Macfarlane. Consequently, she was unable to help women who had the greatest need for early detection of cervical cancer.[13] In the late 1930s Catherine Macfarlane and her collaborators mobilized volunteers for a project that aimed to demonstrate the feasibility of visual screening, and, in a later stage, the efficacy of direct elimination of detected cervical lesions.[14] By the time she published the results of this experiment in 1953, however, the Pap smear was already fully used to screen for cervical cancer in the USA.

Screening campaigns based on the Pap smear

The publication of Papanicolaou and Traut's 1941 article about the use of cervical smears for early detection of cervical tumours (see note 5, Chapter 4) was rapidly followed by attempts to apply the newly developed technique to a systematic examination of all women. In the 1950s and 1960s the growing conviction that the majority of abnormal Pap smears detected precancerous lesions in the cervix, then the observation that it is possible to eliminate such lesions, radically changed the aim of screening campaigns. Originally destined to detect cancers at a stage that gave women greater chances of cure, it became a method for preventing a potentially deadly disease. With the shift to prevention, screening for cervical cancer became a public health issue. In some countries the promotion of screening was nevertheless left to the initiative of individual doctors, health educators, and cancer charities. Other countries elected to organize central screening campaigns, often coupled with the active encouragement of women to get screened. The argument in favour of the second approach was that while education works well with middle-class women and their health providers, women who are the most at risk of cervical tumours—those from lower socio-economic strata—are also the ones who are least likely be screened under a voluntary system. An organized screening system is better adapted to deal with social inequalities.

By the late 1940s some US experts were proposing to extend regular Pap smears to all women at risk of cervical cancer (roughly, those between 30 and 60 years of age). Other specialists were not sure, however, whether 'the womanhood of America can be enticed into the laboratory for routine vaginal smears at regular intervals'.[15] The American Cancer Society (ACS), the organization that replaced ASCC after the Second World War, was persuaded that it could be done. One of the main goals of the ACS was to encourage early detection of cancer. The Pap smear was seen as an especially efficient way to advance this goal. In 1948 the ACS sponsored the First National Cytology Conference, and funded training of pathologists by George Papanicolaou. The US National Cancer Institute and the US Public Health Service also energetically promoted use of the Pap smear.

One of the main obstacles to the generalization of cervical smears was the cost of this preventive approach. Reading of cytological preparations is a specialized, labour-intensive, and therefore expensive activity. It is also error-prone. In the 1960s and 1970s some experts hoped that these problems would be solved through the automatization of reading the slides. At that time scientists had developed machines for an automatic analysis of blood cells, and had high hopes that they could adapt these machines to the automatic analysis of cervical smears. These hopes did not materialize (in the twenty-first century scientists are again working on the automatic reading of Pap smears by optical instruments). The generalization of Pap smears became possible thanks to recruitment of numerous cytology technicians (mostly women), who read the cervical smears. The technicians' work was supervised by pathologists (in the 1960s and 1970s, mostly men) who examined abnormal microscope slides and provided a definitive diagnosis. This was a complicated and costly arrangement but it worked. It became the basis of screening for cervical cancer in all Western countries.

When the BECC director Malcolm Donaldson visited the USA in 1950 he was impressed by the cancer-detection clinics, developed by the ACS, and dedicated mainly to screening for cervical cancers. He reported to the BECC that more than 100 such clinics were active in the USA, and that in 1949 they had examined approximately 50,000 women.[16] However, Donaldson believed that commitment to the ideal of equality upheld by the newly founded UK National Health Service (NHS), and high costs of screening for all precluded the development of similar screening clinics in the UK. Donaldson was wrong. A grassroots initiative by a group of women succeeded in persuading the British authorities that national screening for cervical cancer was feasible. At its origins, efforts were made by the British association of women doctors, the Medical Women Federation. The Association of Registered Women Doctors was founded in London in 1879 to promote women in medicine. It changed its name in 1916 to the Medical Women Federation (MWF). The MWF's interest in women's health led to its involvement in the organization of the Women's National Cancer Control Campaign. The idea to start such a campaign emerged at a February 1964 meeting of the Stoke Newington Liaison Committee of the Women's Peace Group. This progressive and anti-militarist group had previously been active in backing the ban on testing nuclear weapons. With the passage of the Test Ban

Treaty, the group was looking for another militant cause. They had heard, partly by chance, that 3,000 women die annually in the UK from an easily preventable disease, and decided to found a committee for the promotion of screening for cervical cancer. The group contacted the MWF, which was immediately interested. A Labour Member of Parliament, Ms Joyce Butler, joined the committee, and put this problem on Parliament's agenda.[17]

The Women's National Cancer Control Campaign was founded in January 1965 and named Joyce Butler its president. The campaign's main sponsor was the MWF, and it had links with numerous organizations, such as the Association for Maternal and Child Welfare, the Women's British Legion, the Family Planning Association, the National Council of Women, the British Society for Clinical Cytology, the Labour Party, and the Communist Party Women's Committee. One of the campaign's first successes was to promote debates on screening for cervical cancer in Parliament. One of the arguments employed in these debates was that introduction of the contraceptive pill may increase cancer risk 'because we are tampering in the dark on a very delicate piece of machinery'.[18] Efficient prevention of gynaecological cancers could diminish such putative danger. Debates on the generalization of Pap smears in the UK focused on the difficulty of recruiting qualified cytology technicians. It was automatically assumed that such technicians would be female, and therefore that it would be necessary to create part-time jobs to allow married women to work in the laboratories. Experts also discussed the frequency of screening (every 5 or every 3 years) and potential problems with false-negative and false-positive results.

Between 1964 and 1966 the number of UK women screened for cervical cancer tripled, as did the number of technicians who read the cervical smears. In 1966 cervical cancer screening was introduced as a national service by the UK government. The NHS created local coordinating committees to implement this measure. However, in 1968 it became clear that the proposed approach—the creation of numerous screening centres—was not working very well. Facilities established at great cost were not fully used, highly skilled technicians were under-employed, and clinics had begun to close. One of the problems was women's lack of confidence in the efficacy of screening. Behaviour that seems 'unreasonable' from a doctor's point of view, such as reluctance to be screened, Dr John Wakefield from the Christie Hospital in Manchester, explained, 'may be perfectly reasonable from the point of view of a outwardly healthy woman who worried about her work, her mortgage, her family, and does not have much faith in doctor's efficacy.'[19]

The concern about the lack of demand for cervical screening blended with the growing concern that women who were most at risk were also those who were least likely to be screened. Many women of lower socio-economic status, with larger families, and migrant women resisted screening and were unable to provide precise reasons why they rejected it. Health educators from around the country began to research how to persuade women to be screened.[20] They concluded that refusal of Pap smears was often associated with the growth of immigration, and began to publish pamphlets and booklets in Hindi, Urdu, and Turkish directed at women from migrant communities. Health authorities also attempted to bring screening to women who needed it most through the development of mobile screening clinics, established in caravans which were parked near major housing estates. Such mobile clinics were, however, expensive to maintain, difficult to clean, and sometimes vulnerable to vandalism.

In addition, many among the women who visited them were interested in treatment of already existing gynaecological problems, not in screening for cancer.

Finally, the British health authorities decided that the most efficient solution was the implementation of Pap screening by GPs under the supervision of public health physicians. In the early 1970s screening for cervical cancer was defined as a community service. Educational leaflets stressed that the Pap smear is a simple, painless procedure, and presented the treatment of cervical lesions as equally unproblematic. Studies that interviewed GPs who performed Pap smears and of women who were screened revealed a more complicated image: the insertion of the speculum was not always painless, GPs were not always familiar with the range of variation in cervical anatomy, some of the samples they obtained were inadequate, and not all doctors were happy to perform this task. Nevertheless, the NHS was able to build a reliable network of GPs, public health doctors, cytology laboratories, gynaecologists, and oncologists. Testing for cervical cancer in the UK never became a truly routine medical practice. It did become, however, a reasonably efficient public health programme.

Persuading women to be tested: British educational films

In the 1960s the Women's National Cancer Control Campaign sponsored short films on screening and early detection of female cancers. Some of these short films, destined mainly to be projected in cinemas, linked the call to undergo Pap smears with the injunction to see a doctor rapidly when noticing suspicious symptoms. These films aimed to promote screening for female cancers among women of lower socio-economic status, and thus to overcome the main perceived obstacle for such screening in the UK. They also aimed to reduce the fear of cancer and to promote the view that it was a curable disease. One way of achieving the latter goal was to blur the difference between the elimination of precancerous lesions of the cervix and the treatment of invasive malignancies.

In the first scenario, 'Calling all women', a young mother, Mrs Jones, has a Pap smear. The film stresses that the insertion of a speculum, an examination that makes women especially anxious, is not painful. Mrs Jones's smear shows suspicious cells, and she undergoes 'cancer treatment'; that is, an excision biopsy. Her doctor explains to her that the cancer is localized in the cervix, and therefore she has an excellent chance of being cured. During her short hospitalization for the procedure, Mrs Jones gets help from a health visitor to cope with her household duties. She is reassured by her physicians that in spite of the treatment she can have children and sex ('it won't make any difference to your married life'). In the last image in this film, the heroine is playing with her children: 'to look at her now, you'd never believe she'd ever had a thing wrong with her, let alone cancer'.

The second film, 'Emergency stop', shows three women on a bus—two in their 30s and a middle-aged woman ('Gran')—with a small boy. Gran is telling them about a friend who luckily went to the clinic in time, and had 'the test'. She explains that the test is so easy, like post natal, and the mother says 'shh, not in front of the boy'. Gran then talks about another friend who was also lucky, because the lump in her breast was found quickly, and she was cured, and adds, 'she is all right, they only kept her a week or so, she says she hasn't felt so well in years'. One of the women adds 'well it must have pulled her down, having that all the time….' The other woman is convinced now to call the clinic immediately and schedule a Pap smear, and she hurries to do it.

The third film, 'Take action', is situated in a factory which employs female workers. One of the workers says that she learned about cancer screening and that they all have to have it. The shop steward, Peg, goes to the (male) plant manager, telling him that other work places, like Marks & Spencer, had organized testing for their female work force. The manager immediately agrees to do the same, and calls the local Officer of Health. The latter explains that in order to send health workers to the plant, they need to organize a full screening session. Peg and friends produce posters and leaflets. They also provide information to men because, 'while they do not get it, they need to be concerned: cancer hits them where it hurts—no more nights out at the pub, no more football on Saturdays, just staying home with all these grizzling kids'. An Indian worker, Amina, volunteers to translate the posters into Hindi. Men, indeed, became concerned, fearing the loss of their spouses to cancer. The screening session is a big success, with 95% attendance.

The main message of the fourth film, 'Cancer control', explains that cervical cancer can ruin a family's life. It shows health visitors interviewing uncooperative men in a working-class neighbourhood. At first the workers resent the 'meddling' visitor. An off voice comments that, 'if a working class "mum" falls ill, the husband has almost no chance of keeping the family together'. The children are either divided between relations or looked after by the local authority. A health visitor adds that if the problem is short term then one can ask neighbours to help. The film switches to an interview with a working-class woman who has undergone screening for cervical cancer. She explains that the test is rapid, and 'a babysitter is easy to arrange'.

The fifth film, 'The building site', stresses that men should also be concerned about screening for cervical cancer. It shows a worker coping with a large family while his wife spends a few days in hospital following a positive Pap smear. His mates are making fun of him, until they realize that it could happen to them too. They start asking questions about the test, and the worker whose wife is being treated explains how happy he is that his wife is doing well and is going to be fine. He ends by saying 'if you want to know any more, get your old woman to go to the clinics'.

In the sixth film, 'Over the wall', three women are chatting over the garden wall. One of the women had a Pap smear after the birth of her last child and persuades a second woman, who is pregnant, that it is not a big deal. The third women has no children and thinks that she does not need to be concerned by this test, but the other women inform her that this is not the case. The three women then discuss one of their neighbours who had a positive Pap smear, was treated at the local hospital, and who will come back home soon. They also mention one of their friends whose husband at first was opposed to 'the test'. A health visitor who tried to convince him failed at first, but she found an unexpected ally: the husband of the woman who tested positive and was treated successfully. The latter was going to persuade his mate to get his wife to be tested.

The last film, 'Stay young, stay with us', incorporated the call to be screened for cervical cancer into a more general message on the importance of prevention. A girl who got married in her teens faces multiple disasters because she has not heard about prevention. The water pipes in her house burst, she sets accidentally fire to a neighbouring house without being insured, and her children are not vaccinated and have to be put in quarantine.

Finally she reforms, and takes all the necessary preventative actions, including a test for cervical cancer, which will keep her healthy.

The 1960s UK educational films convey an infallibly upbeat message: tests are simple and easy, and even if a positive result is found, it is not a big cause for concern. A short stay in hospital will solve the problem and give women the certainty of good health in the future. They also stress that screening saves the lives of mothers of young children, implicitly affirming that a mother's responsibility to her children includes screening herself for cervical cancer. If they neglect such screening their children may end up in an orphanage. The UK Women's National Cancer Control Campaign aspired to reduce cervical cancer deaths among working-class women, who were especially endangered by this disease, and devised educational materials specifically directed at these women. Similar films made in the USA stressed the role of screening in providing freedom from the threat of cancer, and increasing personal happiness. They did not put to the fore the mother's responsibility for her children, and did not attempt to redress inequalities in access to medical information.

Debates on optimal screening

Once the specialists adopted the principle of screening for cervical cancer, the next question was what age such screening should start, at what age it should stop, and how often should it be done. Countries with national and regional screening programmes usually propose the start of screening at 25, and continue it to the age of 65. After the death of Jade Goody some UK activists campaigned for screening from age 20. Public health experts opposed this idea. Epidemiological data, they argued, showed that Jade Goody was an exception. Very few young women develop cervical malignancies, and those who do tend to have rapidly growing tumours, difficult to spot through regular screening. Moving the start of screening from age 25 to 20 would be inefficient and would produce more harm than good. The proposal to reduce the age of first screening was finally rejected.

Young women seldom develop cervical cancer. By contrast, older women may suffer from this disease, although it is more frequent in the middle-aged. The decision to stop screening for cervical cancer at the age of 65 was justified by the observation that cervical lesions usually evolve very slowly. This is especially true in older women. The elimination of such lesions in women in their late 50s and early 60s should protect them until they reach their late 70s and 80s, an age at which they may have multiple health problems, and the small additional risk of cervical cancer will probably not be their greatest worry. Not all specialists agree. In the USA, in absence of uniform national rules on screening, some doctors continue to give Pap smears to women in their 70s.

Epidemiologists who modelled the growth of cervical lesions proposed that women with two or three consecutive negative Pap smears should be tested only every 3 years. This principle was adopted officially by the World Health Organization (WHO).[21] Some experts, especially in the USA, contested the WHO rules. Jerome Groopman, professor at the Harvard Medical School, explained that Pap smears are notoriously inaccurate. Even under optimal conditions—well-prepared slides, well-trained and alert cytology technicians—the test fails to detect approximately a quarter of abnormal changes in the cervix. Luckily, the high frequency of tests compensates for the high proportion of errors. A yearly Pap smear improves women's chances of escaping cancer.[22] A 2004 editorial in *Diagnostic Cytology* similarly criticized recommendations to increase the interval between Pap smears. Such recommendations will save money for health insurers, but will decrease the quality of women's care:

> investment in annual cervical cancer screening is in many ways like investing in diversified funds for the long term: not very exciting but a very effective way to lower your risk of cancer over a lifetime.... It is important for women investing in their own health to have their investment choices appropriate for their goals of cervical cancer prevention for their entire life, and not just one 3-year window in time. A more efficient but less effective Pap test may not be the best way to meet these investment goals.[23]

The proposal that more is always better was vigorously criticized by other specialists, especially those concerned by the collective aspects of screening. Screening for cervical cancer, undoubtedly efficient in principle, may nevertheless be inefficient in practice. Some women may be over-screened, and suffer from the negative effects of false-negative results and unnecessary diagnostic tests, while other women may be under-screened, because they are unable to obtain access to appropriate health services. Moreover, screening for cervical cancer is not a goal in itself. It is equally important to ascertain that all the women with positive Pap smears undergo further evaluation and have access to quality treatment.[24]

An exemplary success story?

In the early twenty-first century cervical cancer is relatively rare in Western countries, including those with imperfect screening programmes. Fewer than 10 Western women in 100,000 develop this disease every year, and 2 to 4 in 100,000 die from it. The mortality from this disease is much lower than from other cancers, such as lung, colon, or breast. For example, in 2009 2.4 British women per 100,000 died from cancer of the cervix, as compared with 32.0 from lung cancer, 26.2 from breast cancer, 14.0 from colon cancer, 9.7 from ovarian cancer, and 7.8 from cancer of the pancreas.[25] Once the primary cause of cancer death among women, cervical cancer is no longer counted among the most prevalent malignancies.

The drastic decline in the frequency of this disease has been attributed to the improvement in treatment—better surgical techniques, more precise radiation therapy, and, more recently, the introduction of chemotherapy—but above all it is a result of the generalization of screening for cervical lesions.[26] There is no doubt that the elimination of a precancerous cervical lesion reduces the probability that the treated woman will develop cervical cancer. The reasons for the reduction in the overall frequency of this disease in Western Europe and North America may be somewhat more complicated. Screening for cervical cancer, nearly all the experts agree, has played a role in decreasing mortality from this disease in the West. It is less clear how important this role was. A steady decrease in mortality from cervical cancer started well before the generalization of screening for cervical cancer in the last third of the twentieth century. By 1927 the statistician Janet Lane-Claypon had observed that 'the death rate from uterine cancer has now a downward trend', and added that 'effort should be made for maintaining or accelerating that fortunate trend'.[27]

In the 1970s Scandinavian countries had relatively high rates of cervical cancer as compared to other Western countries. The occurrence of cervical cancer was reduced to a much lower level in 2000. This result was attributed to the implementation of efficient screening programmes. On the other hand, France did not have a national screening programme until 2003, and even after the introduction of this programme the diffusion of the Pap smear, through gynaecologists and GPs, remained imperfect. In 2006 35% of French women had never undergone a Pap smear (as compared with 7% in the USA), while many others—more educated women, those living in cities, those followed by a gynaecologist rather than a GP—had received too many tests according to WHO criteria. Nevertheless, the frequency of cervical tumours in France in 2006 was similar to that in countries with more efficient screening programmes and those which made sustained efforts to reach women from less privileged socio-economic strata.

Elements such as better hygiene, the use of oral contraceptives, changes in sexual behaviour, or other, still unknown variables, might have contributed to the decrease in frequency of cervical tumours in the late twentieth century.[28] There is an intriguing parallel between the decline in frequency of cervical malignancies—a cancer that is linked today with the presence of an infectious agent, the human papilloma virus (HPV)—and a parallel decline in the occurrence of stomach cancer, another malignancy linked with an infectious agent, the bacterium *Helicobacter pylori*. In the early twentieth century stomach cancer was high on the list of deadly tumours, and the greatest cause of cancer death in men. The important decrease in frequency of stomach cancer in Western Europe and North America (but not in other parts of the world) was described as an 'unplanned triumph'.[29] It was attributed to lifestyle changes: the generalization of refrigeration, banning of certain food additives, greater consumption of fresh vegetables, and other, still unidentified elements.

It is possible that even in the absence of any intervention from health professionals the occurrence of cervical cancer in Western countries would have continued to decline, and would have been described as another 'unplanned triumph'. On the other hand, even if the precise extent of the contribution of screening for cervical cancer to changes in occurrence of this disease is unknown, few people question today the efficacy of this preventive measure. Screening campaigns are rightly credited with saving women's lives. An individual benefit for the small percentage of Western women who successfully escaped a cervical tumour thanks to timely elimination of a cervical lesion has, however, a collective price. It may change the sense of body and self of numerous women who do not personally benefit from this screening and who follow a distressing medical trajectory without being at risk of cancer, or, alternatively, receive an uncertain diagnosis such as atypical squamous cells of unknown significance (ASCUS), and remain suspended between health and disease.

The incontestable success of screening for cervical cancer does not exempt this public health intervention from a critical scrutiny. Such scrutiny may become even more important in the twenty-first century. The recent redefinition of cervical cancer as a disease produced by a sexually transmitted virus led to the introduction of tests for the presence of this virus and manufacture of a vaccine which is expected to protect against it. These developments may drastically alter screening for cervical malignancies. Nevertheless, it is unlikely that they will eliminate all the complex problems linked with such screening.

6

CERVICAL CANCER BECOMES A SEXUALLY TRANSMITTED DISEASE

Nuns, mothers, and cancer of the womb

In the early nineteenth century physicians proposed numerous and often contradictory theories on the origins of cancer of the womb. This disease was linked by some doctors with sexual excesses and immorality. 'Lower class women who live in cities', the Canadian doctor Guilliame Vallée explained in 1826, 'are decidedly more affected [by uterine cancer] than those who live in the countryside…and how can one explain such a difference if not by their greater moral laxity?'[1] Other physicians noted, however, that prostitutes did not seem to suffer from uterine tumours more often than 'honest' women did. The long list of suspected causes of tumours of the womb included masturbation, excessive sexual activity, syphilis and other venereal diseases, celibacy and sexual abstinence, sterility, great sadness, excessive mourning, dangers of urban life, fright, sequelae of childbirth, abortion, and disorders of women's 'critical age' (menopause). Some nineteenth-century doctors proposed that this disease was more frequent among lower-class women, others claimed that it was often found among upper-class women, and more still that it was more frequent at both extremes of the social spectrum. These debates could only be settled by the collection of quantitative data.

In 1842 a surgeon from Padua, Italy, named Domenico Rigoni-Stern gave a talk at the Fourth Congress of Italian Scientists on 'Statistical facts relative to the disease of cancer'. In this talk, later published as an article, Rigoni-Stern affirmed that nuns rarely suffered from cancer of the womb.[2] Domenico Rigoni-Stern was a pioneer of the statistical approach to the study of cancer, and was especially interested in cancers of the breast and uterus. Some authors argued later that he had uncovered the link between sexual relations and cervical cancer. This is inaccurate. Rigoni-Stern did not claim that nuns were free from uterine tumours. He only stated that this disease was less frequent among nuns than among married women. His aim was to point out an intriguing contrast between the relative rarity of uterine tumours among nuns and the high frequency of breast cancer in this group.

The observation that nuns had a tendency to develop breast tumours was not new. The Italian physician Bernandino Ramazzini (1633–1717) had commented in 1713 on the fact that nuns often suffered from malignant tumours of the breast.[3] The French historian Jacques Le Brun collected the stories of eighteenth-century nuns who suffered for many years from open, suppurating breast lesions that had literarily 'eaten' their chest. Stoical suffering of nuns with malignant, but slow-growing, tumours of the breast was presented as an edifying example of Christian attitude to pain, but also as a display of their deep identification with Christ's wounds.[4] There were no similar examples of stoical suffering of nuns with cancer of the womb. The observation that the same group of women had an unusually high rate of one kind of female cancer, and an unusually low rate of other female malignancy, challenged the popular claim that some people had a hereditary predisposition to malignant tumours. Domenico Rigoni-Stern's observations hinted that cancer is not a single disease, and that different cancers may have distinct causes.

A British physician J.C.W. Lever had earlier made a similar observation. Lever observed 120 cases of cancer of the uterus and concluded in 1839 that cancer of the womb was relatively rare among single women: 'Single women bear a proportion of 5.83 per cent., married women 86.6 per cent., and widows 7.5 per cent., affording a complete refutation of the statement, that celibacy favours the development of the disease.'[5] This conclusion, like Rigoni-Stern's data, strengthened the link between sexual relationships and uterine tumours. In the second half of the nineteenth century this potential link was either interpreted as the consequence of excessive sexual activity or, increasingly, as the result of multiple pregnancies. Women who had many children, gynaecologists had observed, were especially prone to this disease. Occasionally cancer of the uterine cervix was observed in virgins and in childless married women, but the great majority of women who died from uterine tumours had had several children.

In the late nineteenth and early twentieth centuries, when doctors differentiated cancer of the cervix from that of corpus uteri, they noticed that only cervical cancer was linked with marriage and childbirth. Louisa Garrett Anderson and Kate Platt's 1908 data on patients treated for cancer of the womb at the London New Hospital for Women indicated that cancer of the cervix was mainly found in younger women and in those with children: 'in the cervix cases, the average age of the patients was 44.5 years, and the average number of children per patient was five, while 107 women [half of their sample] had had five or more children.'[6] By contrast, cancer of corpus uteri developed as a rule later in life, and was as frequent in childless women as in those who had given birth. These data hinted that cancer of the cervix and cancer of the uterine body were different diseases.

Trauma of childbirth and malignant tumours

Until the mid twentieth century doctors believed that pathological scarification of tears in the cervix produced by childbirth favoured the development of uterine tumours. In the nineteenth and early twentieth centuries doctors believed that cancer was produced by chronic irritation. Such irritation could be the result of persistent inflammation (e.g. presence of an abscess that refused to heal) or the consequence of prolonged contact with an irritating substance. In 1775 the British surgeon Percival Pott (1713–1788) described cancer of the scrotum in chimney sweeps in London, and linked it with chronic irritation of the scrotum by soot. In the early twentieth century doctors observed cancers in workers who handled substances such as tar, asbestos, or aniline dyes, and similarly explained the development of these cancers by chronic irritation by these chemical substances.

Cancer was also linked to irritation produced by chronic burns. In the late nineteenth century British doctors had observed a high frequency of aggressive skin cancer in the valley of Kashmir in India. People in that region warmed their body with a 'Kangri basket'—a mud container filled with coals and enclosed in a basket made of willow—which was kept under their clothes in the winter. People who used Kangri baskets often suffered from chronic burns and ulcers. Sometimes these burns led to the development of a specific form of skin cancer, called Kangri burn cancer, a disease still present among poor people in Kashmir.[7] Egyptians who carried near the skin small metal flasks filled with hot cinders suffered from a similar type of tumour, the 'Cairo burn cancer'. Cancers observed in scientists and technicians who worked with X-ray equipment or manipulated radium were at first explained by the fact that X-rays and radium produced burns. Only from the mid twentieth century onwards were these cancers attributed to mutations—changes in the hereditary material of the cell—induced by radiation.

The irritation theory for the origins of cancer was consolidated in the second half of the nineteenth century when cancer was defined as an abnormal proliferation of cells. Chronic inflammation or permanent irritation of tissues usually leads to a rapid proliferation of cells. Such proliferation, scientists believed, may sometimes become a permanent feature of a given tissue. Cells may lose their ability to stop their division, become aggressive, and end by invading other tissues. The same putative mechanism—a quick proliferation of a group of cells—could explain links between mechanical trauma and cancer. A trauma often leads to the formation of a rapidly multiplying scar tissue. In that case too, scientists believed, some cells may escape control mechanisms and became eternally proliferating, aggressive entities. The latter mechanism could also explain why women who had many children were more vulnerable to cervical cancer. These women suffered more frequently from tears and lacerations of the cervix, and thus from a mechanical trauma which, the German physician and pioneer of the cellular theory, Rudolf Virchow, proposed in 1863, favoured the development of cancer of the womb.

Putative links between cancer of the uterus and pathological scarification of laceration of the cervix could also explain why this disease was found more often in women from lower socioeconomic strata. Poor women had more children. They also had no means to receive proper care, even very elementary care, when they gave birth.[8] In addition, poverty was linked with poor hygiene. Women who had difficulty maintaining a good level of personal cleanliness were more prone to chronic inflammation of the cervix, seen as an additional irritating element. Finally, women from the lower classes suffered more frequently from gynaecological diseases, including sexually transmitted ones, had more abortions, miscarriages, and were more often in poor general health; these are all conditions that were believed to increase the chances of developing cancer of the womb.

Sexuality was not entirely absent from the argument on links between poverty and cervical tumours, since sexually transmitted diseases and abortions were related to the supposedly more lax sexual mores of lower-class women. Nevertheless, in the first half of the twentieth century the majority of experts believed that a higher occurrence of cervical cancer among poor women was mainly the result of frequent pregnancies, inadequate medical care, and harsh life conditions. Cervical cancer was not presented any more as a direct consequence of an immoral life, but rather as a scourge which disproportionately and unfairly affected working-class mothers. This image, we have seen, was still prevalent in British educational films produced in the 1960s.

Race, circumcision, and cervical cancer

Social conditions and factors such as the number of children were but one way to account for variation in the occurrence of cervical tumours. A competing explanation was hereditary susceptibility. Frederick Hoffman (1865–1946), a statistician of the Prudential Insurance Company, one of the pioneers of medical statistics in the USA, and the author of a monumental study on *Race Traits and Tendency of the American Negro* in 1896, published a book that affirmed (one may add, on the basis of rather limited data) that cervical cancer is more frequent among US black women than among white ones.[9] He might have related this observation to differences in income, status, and number of children. Black women often had numerous children, lived in poor hygienic conditions, had fewer chances to receive appropriate medical care when they gave birth, and were more prone to gynaecological infections. Hoffman was persuaded, however, that the main difference between white and black women was not life conditions, but a presumed 'racial susceptibility'.

Black women were reported to have a higher than average frequency of cervical cancer. Jewish women were found to be less susceptible to the disease. From 1901 onward, some doctors claimed that Jewish women had especially high rates of breast cancer and especially low rates of cervical cancer. The first supposition was not confirmed by quantitative studies. Janet Lane-Claypon, among others, observed selected Jewish families with an unusually high occurrence of breast cancer.[10] She was, however, unable to show that Jewish women as a group were more prone to breast cancer than non-Jewish ones.[11] By contrast, several quantitative studies indicated that two cancers of the genital organs, cancers of the penis in men, and cancer of the cervix in women, were relatively rare among Jews. Some cancer experts, such as the US specialist Clarence Little (1888–1971), explained the lower occurrence of cervical cancer among Jewish women by 'racial immunity'.[12] Other specialists linked low rates of cervical cancer among Jewish women and of cancer of the penis among Jewish men with circumcision. Still others proposed that Jewish women may also be protected by their observation of ritual bath prescriptions. One of the main advocates of the circumcision theory, the leading British surgeon and cancer expert Sampson Handley (1872–1962), claimed that other populations practising circumcision, like the natives of Fiji, also had lower rates of cervical cancer than other people in the same area.[13] A Jewish German doctor named Georg Wolff contested these findings. He believed that if one made the appropriate correction for age, life style, social class, and access to doctors (and therefore arrived at an accurate diagnosis) the overall occurrence of cancer of the cervix in Jewish populations was similar to that in non-Jewish ones. The difference, if any, between Jews and Gentiles, may have reflected familial rather than racial differences:

> it may be that a study of heredity will bring us to clearer conclusions, and to tracing the course of events in particular 'cancer families', an important but very difficult piece of work. This, however, is a totally different problem from that of a racial ideology which has but little in common with the exact study of inheritance.[14]

After the Second World War, with the discredit of racial theories, 'racial susceptibility to cancer' was laid to a rest. The question of possible links between circumcision and cervical cancer remained open, however. When scientists showed that a virus transmitted through sexual relations plays a role in the development of cancer of the cervix, this question was redefined as a possible role of circumcision in preventing the of spread of this virus. Circumcision was shown to partially protect men (but not women) from infection by the human immunodeficiency virus

(HIV), the virus which induces AIDS. A 2002 epidemiological investigation concluded that when a man had multiple female sexual partners, circumcision also reduced the risk of cervical cancer for those partners.[15] On the other hand, such reduction was observed only for partners of men with numerous sexual partners and especially risky sexual behaviour, not the most plausible explanation for low rates of cervical cancer observed in the early twentieth century in orthodox Jewish communities. A recent epidemiological study confirmed a relatively low frequency of cervical cancer among Jewish Israeli women. It had also found differences in the occurrence of this cancer between Jewish women of different geographic origins (Europe, North Africa, Yemen). The authors of this study believe that the most probable explanation of their findings was that, 'the low incidence of cervical cancer in Jewish women is genetically determined', probably by hereditary difference in susceptibility to cancer-inducing viruses.[16] The 'racial susceptibility' hypothesis came back, this time associated with a viral explanation for the origins of cervical malignancies.

From irritation, to mutation, to infection

In the era following the Second World War the irritation theory of origins of cancer was gradually replaced by linking cancer to mutations; that is, changes in the hereditary material of the cell. The idea that cancer cells underwent a mutation was not new. It was proposed in the interwar era by geneticists such as Hermann Muller (1890–1967). It was also advocated by some physicians. The British surgeon and cancer expert John Percy Lockhart-Mummery (1875–1957) proposed in 1932 that the common denominator between all the 'irritating' substances credited with the ability to produce malignant tumours was their capacity to induce mutations. Before the Second World War this was, however, a minority view. Nearly all cancer experts adopted variants of the irritation theory. The mutation theory of cancer origins became popular when scientists observed a sharp rise in the frequency of malignant tumours in survivors of the Hiroshima and Nagasaki atomic bombs, and then a similar rise in cancer frequency in animals and humans in nuclear weapons test zones in the Pacific. From the 1940s on, chemical substances such as tar, physical phenomena such as radiation, and biological compounds such as hormones were no longer perceived as powerful 'irritants' that stimulated rapid and uncontrolled proliferation of tissues, but as substances or activities that produced mutations.

The gradual phasing out of the irritation theory of origins of cancer weakened the link between childbirth, lacerations of the cervix, and cervical tumours. In the 1950s and 1960s gynaecologists had noted that childless, sexually active women suffered from cervical cancer. The important element, they then proposed, may not be the number of children but variables such as age of first sexual relationships and the number of sexual partners.[17] At that time, epidemiologists already suspected that 'sexual commerce' may increase the chances of transmission of an infectious agent. In 1974 an article was published in *The Lancet* entitled 'Cancer of the cervix: a sexually transmitted infection?'[18] A 1975 US study concluded that 'cervical cancer has certain characteristics of a venereal disease; in particular the risk has been associated with sexual promiscuity'.[19] Studies of the role of the 'male factor' in the origins of cervical tumour reinforced the infectious hypothesis. Monogamous women married to a man who had had many sexual partners, these studies had shown, had a higher chance of developing cervical cancer than those whose lived with a man who had had only one or two sexual partners.[20]

A viral hypothesis of the origins of cancer was first proposed in the early twentieth century. One of the first advocates of the viral hypothesis was the pathologist Peyton Rous (1879–1970) from the Rockefeller Institute, New York. Rous described in 1910 a virus that induced leukaemia in chickens. The enthusiastic reception of Rous's finding was followed by a hiatus. For a long time researchers failed to uncover similar viruses in human cancers. However, in the 1960s and 1970s they did find viruses associated with rare human cancers such as Burkitt's lymphoma. Moreover, virologists described mechanisms which allowed a virus to remain hidden in the genetic material of a normal cell. Such hidden viruses were suspected of being the cause of numerous human cancers. One of the main aims of the National Cancer Act, signed by US president Richard Nixon in 1971, and known as the War on Cancer act, was to investigate the role of viruses in producing malignant tumours in humans. This goal was not achieved. Scientists did not observe viruses that induced common human cancers, such as breast, colon, or lung. On the other hand, studies funded by the War Against Cancer programme favoured the development of new methods to study viruses. These methods facilitated in turn the investigation of diseases such as AIDS and cervical cancer.

In the 1970s virologists started to look for a 'cervical cancer virus'.[21] The first candidate was the herpes simplex virus (HSV), which induced a sexually transmitted disease. Scientists were unable, however, to find HSV in biopsy material from cervical tumours.[22] A second candidate was cytomegalovirus, another virus that spread through sexual contact. Finally, in 1976 the German virologist Harald zur Hausen (born in 1936) linked cervical cancer with viruses which produced genital warts (warts are benign tumours). Zur Hausen's first candidate was the condyloma virus. Later he and his colleagues amended their original claim and proposed that the probable culprit was another wart-producing virus, the human papilloma virus (HPV).[23] In 2008 zur Hausen was awarded the Nobel Prize in Physiology or Medicine for his discovery of links between HPVs and cervical cancer; he shared the prize with Françoise Barré-Sinusi and Luc Montagnier, who received it for the observation that HIV causes AIDS.

Papilloma viruses were among the earliest viruses linked with cancer in animals. A researcher at the Rockefeller Institute in New York, Richard Shoppe (1901–1966), had found that a papilloma virus produces warts in rabbits. In 1935 Shoppe, who at that point collaborated with the pioneer of studies into the role of viruses in cancer, Peyton Rous, had found out that the rabbit papilloma virus can also produce cancerous growths. In the 1930s Shoppe and his colleagues were unable to show that papilloma viruses are present in cancer cells. In the 1980s, thanks to the development of new molecular biology methods scientists who analysed tissues from women with cervical malignancies demonstrated that they contain HPV. They also showed that cancer was mainly associated with two HPV strains, 16 and 18. Other strains produced benign genital warts, but not cancer.[24] Cervical cancer had begun a new stage in its history: that of sexually transmitted disease.

HPV infection: 'promiscuity' or poverty?

Scientists had shown that the great majority of women with cervical tumours, or with an abnormal proliferation of cervical cells (dysplasia), are infected with HPV. This does not mean, however, that all the women infected with these viruses will develop cancer. Infection by HPV is very common, especially in young women starting their sexual life. In the majority of infected women such an infection usually disappears after a few years (or, to be more precise, the virus cannot be found any more in their cells and secretions). In some women, however, infection by a carcinogenic (cancer-inducing) strain of HPV does not go away. Such persistent infection increases their risk of developing precancerous lesions and malignant tumours. It is not clear why this happens to some women and not to others. Multiple sexual partners at a young age and an early age of first childbirth are associated with greater risk of an infection by a cancer-inducing strain of HPV. Once cervical cancer was redefined as a sexually transmitted disease the links between social class and cervical cancer were attributed—again—to differences in sexual mores. In the 1980s, as in 1826, this disease was linked with a 'greater moral laxity'—or, in today's terms, 'promiscuity'—of women from lower social classes.

The promiscuity hypothesis may, however, be problematic. Before the sexual revolution of the 1960s and 1970s, young women from 'good families' were not expected to have premarital sex and multiple sexual partners. Not all the women respected these rules, but in the 1960s and 1970s epidemiologists assumed that, on average, young women from lower social strata started their sexual life earlier and had more sexual partners than those from a middle-class background.[25] After the sexual revolution of the 1970s the 'promiscuity' hypothesis had lost much of its explanatory value. Many middle-class girls also started their sexual lives early and had numerous sexual partners. The age of first maternity remains, however, a class-related variable: middle-class girls tend to have children later. A more recent epidemiological study found out that Brazilian adolescent girls with precancerous cervical lesions did not have more sexual partners than those without such lesions, on average, and did not start their sexual life earlier. The only important difference between the two groups was the number of pregnancies, which were much higher in the group with premaligant lesions: 'with each additional gestation the adolescents had approximately twice the odds of HISL [a premalignant lesion of the cervix]'.[26] The dangerous combination may be an early start to one's sexual life and early pregnancies. Experts agree that women of lower socio-economic status are at higher risk of cervical cancer, but it is not certain that the only possible interpretation of this observation is the supposition that they are more promiscuous than middle-class women.

The confused experience of HPV infection

Only a small portion of women infected with cancer-inducing HPV strains will develop cancer of the cervix, and in the great majority of these women HPV infection will not produce any harm. Nevertheless, many women view a diagnosis of a carcinogenic strain of HPV as a disturbing and potentially threatening event. Such a diagnosis adds therefore an additional layer of complexity to the already complicated testing for cancer risk. Infection with a dangerous strain of HPV may be likened to the presence of atypical squamous cells of unknown significance (ASCUS), discussed in Chapter 4. But there is one important difference. In the twenty-first century the diagnosis of a persistent infection with a carcinogenic strain of HPV is sometimes interpreted as a judgement on a woman's sexual mores.

Links between sexuality and cervical cancer are at the same time explicit and, to some extent at least, a taboo subject. For example, press articles that discussed the disease and the death of Jade Goody seldom mentioned relationships between sexual relationships and positive Pap smears. The public debate on change in the age of screening for cervical cancer that followed Goody's death was focused on lowering the age of screening for all UK women. Advocates of earlier screening did not propose a specific targeting of young women at higher-than-average risk of cervical malignancy. In Victorian Britain, we were often told, death was omnipresent, and sex was taboo, while in the twenty-first century the opposite is true: sex is everywhere and death has become invisible. The media's treatment of Jade Goody's disease may point to a different direction. We may still be Victorians after all.[27]

The cancer expert and medical writer Jerome Groopman described the dilemmas linked with HPV diagnosis. Jenny, a daughter of a friend of Groopman's, received a positive result from a Pap smear. A follow-up test revealed that she was infected with a carcinogenic HPV strain. A healthy college student, Jenny was stunned and frightened by this result, seen as a veiled threat of cancer. She also felt distressed because she had caught a sexually transmitted infection: 'after a long pause, she told me she had informed the college doctor that she had had intercourse with only two partners in her life, and never without a condom. She added that the doctor had met her statement with a sceptical look'. 'I didn't like his attitude', Jenny said. 'He made me feel as if I must be promiscuous'. Jenny felt obliged to inform her boyfriend about her infection, since HPV put him at an increased risk of penile cancer. He had then found out that he was infected with the same strain of HPV virus. Jenny and her boyfriend hoped that their infection would disappear spontaneously and their HPV tests would soon became negative. Groopman added, however, that a negative test does not necessarily mean that the person is totally virus-free:

> experts now believe that, as with herpes, once you are infected with papilloma, you are infected for life. There is no treatment. In many cases, an active infection is controlled by the immune system and becomes dormant. No one can predict whether, or when, the virus will become active again.[28]

Lisa Spinelli, who writes for the *Boston Phoenix*, provided a vivid description of a life in the shadow of HPV infection and uncertain results of Pap smears and cervical biopsies. The title of her article, 'Living with HPV: it afflicts millions, yet no one talks about this nightmarish sexually transmitted disease', summarizes its content. Lisa Spinelli's problem started when a routine Pap smear diagnosed low-grade abnormal cells. The doctor at the Planned Parenthood Clinics she attended recommended watchful waiting. Spinelli was, however, worried and decided to undergo a colposcopy. The test confirmed that she had cervical lesions. Although her gynaecologist reassured her that only a very small portion of women with this kind of lesion develop cancer, the frequent mention of the disease scared her, and made her tense during the month-long wait for biopsy and HPV test results. She then found out she was infected with a carcinogenic strain of HPV.

The results of the HPV test increased Spinelli's anguish. She decided to fight her fears of cancer through the adoption of a healthy lifestyle. She also decided to stop smoking. The latter decision, one may add, was not merely a health fad: smoking increases the risk of cervical cancer. A year later, her colposcopy results were normal, although her Pap smear still showed low-grade abnormal cells. She fervently hoped the Pap smear results too would became normal soon, but just the opposite happened: she developed vaginal bleeding and was diagnosed with high-grade abnormal cells. Spinelli was scheduled for an electrosurgical excision of her lesions, a procedure she especially dreaded, fearing that it would diminish her chances of becoming pregnant. Finally, after more tests and biopsies, her doctors decided that she was not in immediate danger of cervical cancer and could postpone the surgical elimination of her lesions. Writing in 2009, Lisa Spinelli was not sure whether her problems were truly over or if she was heading for another round of uncertain results and emotional havoc. For her,

> the most debilitating aspect of HPV is not the pelvic ache or cramping, the incredibly uncomfortable scooping and scraping inside or outside your most sensitive parts, or even the waiting for results to determine if you have cancer. It's having no … clue what's coming at you next.[29]

HPV is yet another hidden element of the body which, when it is made visible by new medical technologies, changes the way women feel about their bodies. Like the presence of abnormal cells in a cervical smear, HPV testing has the potential to transform people's everyday attitudes of themselves as primarily healthy, which is taken for granted, to potentially unhealthy. The development of an HPV vaccine was presented by the vaccine's producers as a solution to the dilemma of women who found themselves in such a distressing situation. They would not need to worry about the meaning of a positive test for HPV, because, once vaccinated, their tests would be negative. An new preventive approach would, its promoters claimed, attenuate the problems produced by the previous one.

HPV vaccine: a hard sell

The description of the role of carcinogenic strains of HPV in producing cervical cancer was rapidly followed by the hope of producing a vaccine against these viruses. Several pharmaceutical companies became interested in the manufacture of such a vaccine. Its production, they found, was a complex task. Vaccines against childhood viral disease are based on killed or attenuated virus (the Salk polio vaccine used the first strategy, and the Sabin polio vaccine used the second one). These relatively simple approaches did not work for HPV. Scientists who developed HPV vaccines were obliged to use a complicated genetic engineering technique, the production of virus-like particles (VLPs). The necessity of employing this technique contributed to the vaccine's high price.

Another complex problem was how to test an HPV vaccine. Women infected with HPV develop cancers many years later. Definitive proof that the HPV vaccine reduces the occurrence of invasive cervical cancer is possible to obtain only 15–20 years after vaccination. Such a long delay between the manufacture and the marketing of a product is rarely acceptable for a pharmaceutical firm. In addition, it was not possible for ethical reasons to conduct a randomized, placebo-controlled trial with mortality from cervical cancer as its endpoint. Researchers agreed therefore upon an intermediate proof (a surrogate marker) of the effects of HPV vaccine: reduction in the percentage of women with precancerous lesions of the cervix. Merck, the company that produced the first HPV vaccine Gardasil, compared the percentage of vaccinated and non-vaccinated women who developed such lesions. In 2006 these trials showed that vaccination decreased the frequency of precancerous lesions of the cervix. Gardasil, prepared with four strains of HPV, obtained a US marketing permit in February 2006 and an European one in April 2006.

Merck mounted an important publicity campaign to promote Gardasil's sales and to secure its brandname status before a competing product, the Cevarix vaccine manufactured by GlaxoSmithKline, reached the market (Cevarix was prepared with two strains of HPV, and was granted a marketing permit in 2008). Girls in the USA produced publicity spots singing 'I want to be one less … One less statistic'. One woman said that 'Gardasil is the only vaccine that *may* help protect you against the four types of HPV that may cause 70% of cervical cancer.'[30] The English-language version of this spot stressed girls' choices. The Spanish version put the accent on a mother's role in protecting their daughters.[31] The 'one less' publicity spots for Gardasil focused on an abstract role of a 'virus' in producing cervical cancer, but refrained from mentioning sexual relations and sexual mores. Neither did it mention the complex nature of interactions between HPV and cervical cancer, the role of other risk factors such as early pregnancies or smoking, or the absence (as of now) of proofs of Gardasil's ability to prevent invasive cervical cancer.

The aggressive marketing of the HPV vaccine by its producers was meant to overcome hurdles in its trajectory, such as its high cost and the uncertainty regarding the final results of vaccination. Moreover, to be efficient the HPV vaccine needs to be administered to girls before they become sexually active. This means that parents or educators need to discuss sexually transmitted infection with pre-adolescent girls. This issue was not seen as problematic in Western European countries. In the USA, however, conservative Christians strongly opposed the perceived threat to young girls' innocence, and formed a temporary alliance with feminists who criticized the excessive medication of women's bodies by greedy pharmaceutical companies. In spite of this double opposition, Gardasil became a popular vaccine in the USA.

Vaccination in the USA is made exclusively on a voluntary basis. The majority of US states (with the exception of Virginia) rapidly rejected the possibility of compulsory vaccination, while the US immigration office's 2008 requirement to vaccinate women candidates for immigration was cancelled 2 years later. All Western European countries approved the HPV vaccine, but in 2009 the level of official support for this vaccine varied from one country to another.[32] The costs of the HPV vaccine are entirely covered by the state in the UK, Germany, and Greece, and partly covered in other Western European countries. In the UK and parts of Spain health authorities organized HPV vaccination campaigns in schools, in Denmark, Luxemburg, the Netherlands, and parts of Italy parents received official letters inviting them to vaccinate their daughters, whereas in France, Germany, and Greece the vaccination was made on demand only and the government did not take any special initiatives to promote the vaccine.

In France, the reluctance to organize a vaccination campaign was probably linked with an earlier controversy on vaccination against hepatitis B, another sexually transmitted disease. France conducted in 1980 a mass vaccination campaign of school children against hepatitis B. Several children developed serious neurological side effects attributed to the vaccine. Their parents

sued the French state. In a high-profile process the French government was accused of imprudent haste and collusion with
the pharmaceutical industry (the French firm which produced
hepatitis B vaccine made handsome profits thanks to the mass-
vaccination programme in schools). It is plausible to assume
that the French authorities' decision to abstain from central
directives about vaccination against HPV was influenced by a
wish not to repeat the hepatitis B scandal. However, the exclusive reliance on parental choice strongly privileges the vaccination of middle-class girls. When HPV vaccination is carried out
in schools (as in the UK) 80–90% of preteen girls are vaccinated.
By contrast, on-demand vaccination, even when accompanied by official invitation letters, typically leads to the vaccination of 30–50% of girls. In 2009 the European Cervical Cancer
Association expressed a worry that the HPV vaccine—like the
Pap smear—is mainly used by women who are at the lowest risk
of cervical cancer.

HPV vaccine: many questions, few answers

The HPV vaccine is a promising but problematic preventive
method. Debates about this vaccine were focused on vaccination of boys, short- and long-term efficacy of vaccination, its
effect on the population level, and its potential dangers.

Men are not at risk from cervical cancer, but they are the main
source of HPV infection in women. Those in favour of vaccinat-
ing both sexes argued that since women are infected with HPV
by men it is unfair that only girls face the risks and the cost of vaccination. Vaccination of boys, advocates of this approach added,
would produce herd immunity—the protection of a population
as a whole thanks to the existence of an important number of

individuals who carry antibodies against an infectious agent—and would therefore reduce the overall risk of HPV infection. An additional argument was that men suffer from HPV-related pathologies, such as genital warts. All these arguments were not sufficient to promote the costly vaccination of boys.

The debate on vaccination of boys may be potentially transformed by the recent linking of many head and neck cancers (malignancies which are more frequent in men than in women) with the 'carcinogenic' strains of HPV.[33] The association of HPV infection and head and neck tumours is not new, but scientists had noted an increase in the proportion of HPV-positive head and neck cancers, and found that they are associated with the same HPV strains that induce cervical malignancies. Producers of HPV vaccine may welcome the opportunity to find new users for their product. They may also be unsure how to market their product to these new users. The rise in the number of HPV-positive head and neck tumours is attributed to the growing popularity of oral sex. Producers of anti-HPV vaccines promoted the vaccination of girls without mentioning sexual intercourse. It remains to be seen whether they will be able to promote the vaccination of boys without mentioning oral sex.

The vaccination of (Western) girls was promoted in spite of the persisting uncertainty about the efficacy of HPV vaccine to accomplish its main goal: to protect women from cancer. The mass marketing of an HPV vaccine was made without knowing whether it will ultimately reduce the frequency of cervical cancer. It is not known either how long the anti-HPV immunity will last. A need for periodic re-vaccination may greatly increase the already high costs of the HPV vaccine. Some experts also wonder whether the elimination of cancer-causing strains of HPV will decrease the body's natural immunity to other HPV strains

(strain substitution). If this were the case, it would be necessary to vaccinate girls and women against the new carcinogenic
strains, an endless task. A 2008 editorial in the *New England
Journal of Medicine* asked:

> How can policy makers make rational choices about a medi-
> cal intervention that may do good in the future but for which
> evidence is insufficient, especially since we do not know for
> many years whether the intervention will work or—in the
> worst case scenario—will do harm.[34]

In spite of uncertainties about the long-term efficacy of HPV
vaccine this vaccine is undoubtedly a success, at least for its producers. Aggressive promotion of this vaccine paid off. Merck
and then GlaxoSmithKline made important investments in publicity to non-experts and used skilful lobbying of physicians and
nurses, legislators, and public health administrators. In 2006
hundreds of US doctors and nurses were signed up as unofficial spokespersons for Gardasil. They were trained by Merck,
provided with a multimedia presentation, and paid US$4,500
for each 50-minute talk, delivered over Merck-sponsored meals.
Many were paid for attending Merck 'advisory board' meetings
to discuss the shots. Some experts were paid directly by Merck.
For example, the *New York Times* reported that Gregory Poland, a
vaccine expert at the Mayo Clinic who was a non-voting member
on the US Center for Disease Control panel that recommended
Gardasil in 2006 and then publicly defended the panel's decision, received at least $27,000 in consulting fees from Merck.[35]
In 2008 the Gardasil publicity campaign obtained several US
Pharmaceutical Advertising and Marketing Excellence awards,
and Gardasil was named 'Brand of the Year' by *Pharmaceutical
Executive* magazine.

Some experts who participated in the testing of the HPV vaccine felt that Merck was too aggressive and went too fast. It would have been better, they believed, if the vaccine producers had acted more slowly. But acting slowly was not really a commercially viable option. The full effect of the HPV vaccine on the frequency of cervical cancer is expected to be known in about 20 years, near the time the majority of patents on this product will expire. Manufacturers of the HPV vaccine had to find ways to maximize their investment in this product before it could be proven that it indeed prevents cervical malignancies. The HPV vaccine is a bet on the future, but the bet is made by the vaccine users, not by its producers.

The HPV vaccine is expensive (in 2009 the cost of a three-shot course of Gardasil in the USA was $360) and is not certain to deliver all its promises. Still, it was endorsed by many parents, including those who understood that it is not certain whether the vaccine can prevent cancer. Aggressive promotion of this product undoubtedly contributed to its widespread diffusion, but it may not be the only reason for its commercial success. One of the main benefits of the HPV vaccine will probably be the reduction of the economic and emotional costs of screening and work-up of abnormal Pap smears: close to 3 million such abnormal smears are evaluated yearly in the USA. One of the reasons US parents enthusiastically endorsed Gardasil might have been the wish to spare their daughters the shame, embarrassment, and rocky medical trajectory that may follow diagnosis of an HPV infection. HPV vaccine is also expected to limit the number of distressing ASCUS diagnoses. As the physician and historian of medicine Robert Aronowitz put it:

> the initial construction and marketing of Gardasil as a drug against individual risk for Western markets is not an example of mis-targeting but one which is right on target: Gardasil

promises to reduce this noise in the expensive and wasteful system.[36]

The 'noise-reduction' function is obviously only one of the potential effects of the HPV vaccine. There is a real hope that this vaccine will also reduce the frequency of cervical malignancies, especially in developing countries. These countries are not preoccupied by the harm of screening for cervical cancer—since such screening is often limited or non-existent—but by the high mortality from this disease. The HPV vaccine could be very important in these countries if two conditions are fulfilled: that it prevents cancer and not just precancerous lesions, and that it is sold for a tiny fraction of its original price.

7

STILL A WOMAN'S SCOURGE

Cervical cancer in the global South

In industrialized countries cervical cancer is no longer seen as a major public health problem. Alas, this is not true in other parts of the world. Tumours of the cervix are the first cause of cancer death among women in numerous parts of the world: sub-Saharan Africa, parts of Central and Latin America, and South-east Asia.[1] For example, 49.2% of cancer deaths among women in Haiti are attributed to cervical cancer, as compared with 2.5% in North America.[2] In regard to this disease, as with many other human ailments, the main division is between the West and 'the Rest'. The elevated incidence of cervical cancer in developing countries (from 5 to 10 times higher than in industrialized countries) is attributed to an early age of marriage or cohabitation, multiple sexual partners, multiple pregnancies, early age of first pregnancy, poor genital hygiene, and smoking. Unsurprisingly, developing countries also have much lower rates of cure of cervical cancer. Women are typically diagnosed with more advanced tumours, and receive less efficient treatment. Public health experts believe that relatively modest investments in the prevention of cervical malignancies in developing countries could bring very important health gains. A single cervical smear for all women at age 45 may eliminate a quarter of cervical cancers, and two tests per lifetime at ages 45 and 55 would eliminate 40–45% of these tumours. This seemingly simple goal is, however, often very difficult to put into practice.

High-tech solutions and the naked eye: screening for cervical tumours in resource-poor settings

One of the main problems of screening for cervical lesions in Western countries is the difficulty of reaching women from lower socio-economic strata. It is not too difficult to persuade women to have regular Pap smears when such a smear is a part of a routine gynaecological check up. The goal of screening programmes provided by general practitioners, midwives, or nurses is to reach women who do not see a gynaecologist regularly and to extend screening for cervical malignancies to all women who have contacts with healthcare professionals. But what should one do in places where the majority of women had very limited access to health services? In many regions of the world a screening programme which proposes periodic Pap smears for all women is not a realistic option. Therefore, experts looked for alternatives to the vaginal smear.

One possible solution is a visual examination of the cervix, a screening method proposed by the US physician Catherine Macfarlane in late 1930s. Such an examination can be made by health workers (nurses and nurse-aids) in a regional health care clinic. The health worker uses a speculum to paint the cervix with a 5% solution of acetic acid (the VIA method, visual inspection with acetic acid). Areas of abnormal proliferation appear as white spots on the cervix's surface. Field trials have shown that trained health workers who applied this approach were able to recognize 70–80% of cervical lesions. The specificity of the method (fewer false-positive results) increased when health professionals were instructed to identify only well-defined white zones of the cervix and to neglect the 'intermediate' ones. However, this choice reduced the sensitivity of screening (more false-negative results). It is not clear whether the use of a magnifying lens improved the rate of detection of cervical lesions. Some specialists affirmed that this was the case, and that devices such as a magnavisualizer, an illuminated magnifying glass with two lenses and integrated light, help to identify low-grade cervical lesions. Other experts claimed, however, that the overall efficacy of screening was not helped by such devices, because the advantages of higher sensitivity were cancelled by an increase in the number of false-positive results.

In pilot trials on the efficacy of VIA screening, women with suspected cervical lesions were sent to a clinic for a further investigation and biopsy. Verification of the efficacy of visual screening by trained professionals was important to evaluate the feasibility and the efficacy of VIA. It is not, however, a viable option for mass screening campaigns in resource-poor countries. In these countries public health experts promote the so-called see-and-treat approach. All women with identified cervical lesions are treated on the spot, usually by freezing their lesions with solid carbon dioxide (cryotherapy). The main advantage of the 'see-and-treat' method is that women do not need to return to the clinics, and therefore are not 'lost' to therapy. However, the see-and-treat method has several disadvantages. One is overtreatment. Some women do not need to be treated and suffer unnecessarily from the side effects of cryotherapy. The other is the impossibility of checking whether treatment is justified and efficient. With the see-and-treat approach there are no material elements such as microscope slides or biopsy material that can be examined later to estimate how often the treatment was necessary. Without such verification, health professionals cannot learn from experience and cannot improve their ability to identify dangerous cervical lesions. Finally, some of the women treated for superficial cervical lesions may in fact have invasive tumours, and need more radical therapy.[3]

The see-and-treat method is perceived as an improvement on inaction, but even its most enthusiastic advocates agree that VIA is a less-efficient method for diagnosing cervical lesions than the Pap smear. In the 1970s and 1980s the Pan-American Health Organization (PAHO) strongly supported the introduction of Pap-smear-based screening campaigns in several Latin American countries. The results of these campaigns were ambiguous. The mortality from cervical cancer in countries which implemented such campaigns—such as Mexico, Costa Rica, and Cuba—decreased only slightly, and at the end of the twentieth century was not very different from mortality in neighbouring countries with no screening programmes. A 2001 World Health Organization (WHO) text stated that middle-income countries often propose over-ambitious screening programmes which attempt to cover all women aged 25–60 and to test them all every 3 years. A more realistic approach, WHO experts proposed, would be to focus on a more narrow fraction of women (e.g. those aged 30–50) and give them a single, or at most two good-quality tests in a lifetime. The most important aim of screening programmes should be to reach 80% or more of the targeted women.[4]

In 2007 PAHO experts also recognized that the organization of efficient screening programmes in Latin America is difficult. The PAHO revised its earlier guidelines and recommended the introduction of the see-and-treat approach in Latin America and Caribbean countries, which have a high frequency of cervical cancer and limited possibilities of developing comprehensive Pap-smear-based screening programmes; these countries included Bolivia, Colombia, Guatemala, Peru, Haiti, Honduras, Guyana, and Nicaragua. The PAHO's director, Mirta Roses, explained that if properly implemented the new approach could save thousands of lives:

> We need to bring women into health facilities by having gender-friendly services, by helping them to overcome obstacles in their families and communities, and by not having too many steps in the treatment process. As it is, we too often get women when it is too late, too costly, too painful.[5]

The see-and-treat approach is implemented mainly in so-called middle-income countries. This simplified method of screening is still seen as too expensive for truly poor developing countries. Some specialists hope that the solution for organizing screening for cervical lesions in such countries will not come from the diffusion of low-tech, labour-intensive approaches such as VIA, but, paradoxically, from the newest development in molecular biology. A high-tech method, such as the search for cancer-producing strains of HPV, may be adapted to large-scale use in developing countries. A national screening programme grounded in a visual examination of the cervix needs to train numerous health workers. By contrast, the search for cancer-producing HPV strains can be made by automatic instruments (nucleic acid sequencers) and can be performed in a small number of specialized laboratories. Moreover, women can be taught to prepare for themselves vaginal swabs that are used for the identification of cancer-producing HPV strains. This may eliminate one of the obstacles to the generalization of screening for cervical cancer. Some women are reluctant to undergo a gynaecological examination with a speculum, indispensable for the direct observation of the cervix or the preparation of a cervical smear. A self-sampling method may reduce their unwillingness to be screened. It may also considerably reduce the costs of screening.

A switch from Pap smears to HPV testing was successfully tested in India.[6] The main problem was the low specificity of the test; that is, the high number of false-positive results. Advocates of HPV testing hope to improve its specificity. They also hope that scientists will develop simple and inexpensive kits for diagnosis of HPV strains, reducing the cost of screening even more. Even highly simplified mass-screening programmes cannot work, however, without money, human resources, and a minimal medical infrastructure. The 2001 WHO study stated that,

> In our view, many low-income developing countries, particularly most of those in sub-Saharan Africa, currently have neither the financial and manpower resources nor the capacity in their health services to organize and sustain a screening programme of any sort. Low income developing countries should consider planned investments in order to improve the capacity of their health services to diagnose and treat cervical cancer precursors and early invasive cancers, before considering even limited screening programmes.[7]

Screening for cervical cancer in an 'intermediate' country: Brazilian campaigns

Many regions of sub-Saharan Africa lack even rudimentary health services, and many Latin American countries do not have a public health infrastructure able to deliver preventive health care to lower-class women. This is not the case in Brazil. Many Brazilians are poor. On the other hand, Brazil has world-class hospitals and research facilities, well-trained health professionals, a tradition of public health policy that goes back to the early twentieth century, and a national health service (SUS, or *Sistema Unico de Saude*). In the late 1980s Brazil started an ambitious national programme of screening for cervical cancer grounded in the PAHO's recommendation. This programme, greatly expanded in the early twenty-first century, is successful...sometimes.

Between 1960 and 1980 two models of screening for cervical tumours co-existed in Brazil: colposcopy-based detection and screening based on a Pap smear. Some experts supported the transformation of the so-called triple model—which included coloposcopy, cytology, and, if necessary, cervical biopsy—into a tool of mass screening. Projects such as the Preventive Dispensary of Gynaecological Cancer, in Rio de Janeiro, described in Chapter 4, aimed to persuade health professionals that it is possible to bring the triple method to low-income women. The Red Cross service for the detection of cervical tumours in Belo Horizonte, the capital of the Brazilian state Minas Gerais, was another example of a 'demonstrative project'. This service, opened in 1944, employed a colposcopist and a trained cytologist. Every woman examined underwent a colposcopic examination, a Pap smear, and, if necessary, a biopsy of cervical lesions. The majority of the users of this service were women from the city of Belo Horizonte, but its directors also organized a small screening campaign in a rural area of Minas Gerais, to show that it was possible to provide high-quality colposcopic screening outside big cities.

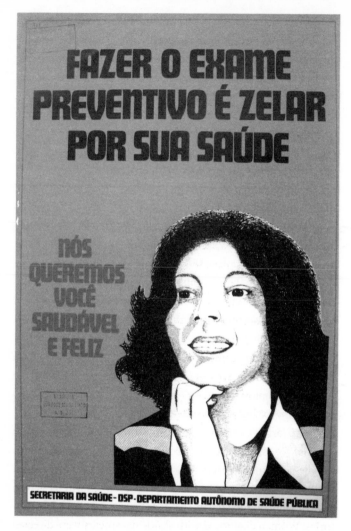

3. Brazilian cervical cancer poster. The poster reads 'Do a preventative test. We want you healthy and happy.'

Museo de Saude Pulica Emilio Ribas, Sao Paolo, Brazil.

In the 1960s and 1970s several small screening campaigns employed colposcopic examination. The organizers of a larger campaign in rural zones of Parana state, conducted in the early 1970s, at first also aspired to propose colposcopical examination for all women who were screened. They found, however, that the exportation of the triple model outside big cities was a complicated endeavour, and settled for a compromise solution. The majority of women had only a Pap smear, but in a few selected localities all screened women also underwent a colposcopical examination. The Parana campaign employed mobile intervention units. In a first stage, three to four physicians were sent to a targeted locality to prepare the ground for the campaign. In a second stage, buses transported 50–60 people—doctors, nurses, secretaries, and social assistants—to that municipality. The mobile units organized screening, educational activities, and standardized collection of data, and left once they had accomplished these tasks, a strategy that facilitated the covering of larger zones of the state's interior.

Other screening campaigns in rural areas of Brazil relied on using the Pap smear. A campaign in Bahia state, conducted in the late 1960s, employed fixed rather than mobile staff, and reserved colposcopy exclusively for women with abnormal Pap smears. Another, larger campaign in Pernambuco state, conducted in the mid 1970s, enrolled approximately 300,000 women in 10 middle-sized municipalities. Each town hosted a screening unit with a physician, a nurse, and a sanitary visitor who collected vaginal smears. Pap smears were read in two reference laboratories. Women diagnosed with abnormal smears were directed to a central cervical pathology clinic in the state's capital for a colposcopic examination and biopsy. The campaign's goal was to screen all eligible women every 2 years.

In the 1960s and 1970s Brazilian public health experts conducted numerous screening campaigns. Official reports of these campaigns presented them as successful endeavours. The reality was often less impressive. Some campaigns had considerable local success, at least for a few years, but they were not able to provide stable and efficient large-scale screening. Even in big cities with multiple screening centres, such as Rio de Janeiro, preventive actions had a modest effect—if any— on the frequency of cervical cancers, the proportion of women diagnosed with advanced, incurable tumours, and mortality from this disease. The situation was decidedly worse outside the major cities. Created in a fragmented manner and applied in a discontinuous fashion, screening programmes destined for Brazil's interior were, as a rule, small-scale enterprises. They often suffered from a shortage of staff, equipment, and funds, and reached only a limited number of women.

In the mid 1970s the growing realization that some parts of Brazil were continuing to have an alarmingly high rate of mortality from cervical cancer, coupled with pressure from the PAHO, increased governmental interest in the prevention of this disease. At that time the support for colposcopy-based programmes waned, and all the new screening programmes relied on Pap smears. In 1973 the Brazilian Health Ministry created the first PAHO-sponsored National Programme of the Control of Cancer. This programme, based in the São Paulo region, promoted the early diagnosis of cervical cancer, training of cytotechnicians, and standardization of cancer registries. Another programme started in the city of Campinas (São Paulo state) then was successfully extended to the entire Campinas region. The official support for large-scale screening campaigns was intensified in the late 1980s, and led to the creation of numerous regional programmes. Still, poor women often did not have easy access to screening. In the mid 1990s women who wanted to get a Pap smear in a public facility in Recife (a town of north-east Brazil with high rates of cervical cancer) faced a true obstacle course:

> in 1994, a woman arriving at the *Hospital de Câncer*'s cervical cancer screening service for the first time realistically needed to be at the hospital by 4 or 5 a.m. in order to insure a place in line in triage. When triage opened at 7 a.m. the woman will be referred to *departmento do pelvis* where she would wait, jammed between a dozen other women in two small rooms, to have her name called to sign a paper that would assure that the hospital would get paid. She would then return to wait to be attended, often standing, anywhere from one to four more hours, leaving at midday or 1 p.m. As she left, the woman would make an appointment, for one or two months hence, to pick up the results of her examination.[8]

In 1995 the Brazilian Institute of Cancer started a national campaign of screening for cervical cancer, named *Viva Mulher* (Life for Women). At first conceived as a pilot project, *Viva Mulher* was implemented in six important Brazilian cities: Recife, Brazilia, Rio de Janeiro, Belém, Curitiba, and Sergipe. In 1998 the Ministry of Health transformed this project into a permanent programme destined to provide triennial Pap smears to all Brazilian women. The ministry also promoted the development of a national computerized database on cervical tumours. The results of the first 10 years of the *Viva Mulher* programme were mixed. The new programme greatly increased the number of screened women and tests performed. The frequency of cervical cancers in poorer regions of Brazil, especially in the north east, remained high, however, and the mortality from this disease was not affected by the impressive increase in the number of Pap smears.[9]

Experts explained the limited success of the *Viva Mulher* programme by the persistence of technical problems, such as poor organization of screening campaigns and errors in the reading of microscopic slides. The frequency of cervical cancers in a given locality, Brazilian public health specialists had proposed, reflected the overall quality of health services in this locality, since, 'cervical cancer is an excellent tracer condition for primary care in general, based on the similarity of such concepts as accessibility, coverage, comprehensiveness, technical and scientific quality, and effectiveness'.[10] The implicit conclusion is that elimination of the technical shortcomings of the existing screening programmes will make them as efficient as those in industrialized countries. Anthropologists who studied health care in Brazil drew a more complex picture, and pointed to the difficulty of dissociating technical obstacles to the introduction of efficient health care measures from broader economic and social problems.

The symbolic life of cervical tumours in north-eastern Brazil

Affluent people in middle-income countries who can afford private health insurance (typically between 10 and 20% of the population) have access to high-quality health care. Others, that is the great majority of citizens, are not merely denied access to some of the services and commodities available to more affluent people, they may also suffer from an inadequate and occasionally harmful use of Western medicine's resources. The US anthropologist Nancy Scheper-Hughes, who studied women's and children's health in a poor area of north-east Brazil, observed the combined effects of insufficient and excessive utilization of drugs and medical services.[11] Poor women had very high levels of caesarean sections and surgical sterilizations, while their children were fed—often in an inappropriate way—formula milk, and received—often unnecessarily—high doses of antibiotics. In spite of an important consumption of medical products and services, mothers and children often suffered from poor health, and many young children died. Some Brazilian health experts explained that the main problem was women's ignorance, and the solution was to teach them to do 'the right thing', for example to breastfeed their babies. Scheper-Hughes had made the persuasive argument that the chaotic use of pharmaceuticals, processed baby foods, and medical procedures was the result of instability and tension in women's lives and their difficult working and living conditions. It also reflected aggressive marketing of 'modern' medical technologies, presented to poor people as an appropriate solution to their problems.

Another US anthropologist, Jessica Gregg, studied attitudes to screening for cervical cancer in a *favela* (shanty town) in Recife. She had found that cervical cancer is entangled in Brazil in a dense network of symbolic meanings, many of which are directly related to the cultural understanding of women's sexuality.[12] In the 1990s, well-intentioned health educators conducted a vast public campaign to teach the *favela* women about the dangers of cervical malignancies and the advantages of prevention. They emphasized the risks of becoming sexually active at a young age, multiple sexual partners, and early pregnancies. Health workers also insisted on the importance of 'prevention'—that is, regular Pap smears—for sexually active women. The campaign's main slogan was '*quem faz sex, faz prevençao*' (roughly 'if you have sex, practice prevention'). This slogan and the campaign's focus on women's (but not men's) sexual activity were problematic, however. They implicitly attributed cervical cancer to women's deviant sexual behaviour, and associated the prevention of this disease exclusively with present-time sexual activity. Cervical cancer is, however, frequent in women over 45. Many of the older women in the *favela* were no longer sexually active, and assumed therefore that they need not concern themselves with screening for this malignancy.

Women interviewed by Jessica Gregg saw the Pap smear as a way to prevent all sexually transmitted diseases. This view was reinforced by health workers who told women that other gynaecological diseases increase the danger of cervical cancer (this is true for HIV infection, but not for banal gynaecological ailments). Women in the *favela* saw the Pap smear as a 'cleansing' procedure that eliminates infections and makes a woman clean inside. This confusion was reinforced by their use of the term *prevençao* as a description for all gynaecological examinations conducted with a speculum, including biopsies for suspected cervical malignancies. It was also strengthened by the fact that doctors and nurses often told to women with cancerous or precancerous conditions that they suffered from 'inflammation', a term which they also used to describe non-malignant gynaecological diseases. For example, a woman diagnosed with cervical cancer explained that she went to the maternity clinics: 'they did *prevençao* there, took a piece out and said that I had an inflammation'.[13]

The precise meaning of cleansing through a Pap smear often reflected the sexual strategy chosen by a given woman to survive in the harsh world of the *favela*. Jessica Gregg observed two kinds of sexual strategy. Some women elected 'security'. They remained faithful to their male partner and accepted his infidelities as a fact of life. These women saw the Pap smear as a way to limit the dangers that stemmed from their partner's lax sexual mores. This test was an 'obligation', forced on them at regular intervals by the irresponsible behaviour of men and uncontrolled sexual drives of other women. Other women elected 'liberty'. They had multiple sexual partners and changed them according to their circumstances and needs. Those women did not view the Pap smear as a regular duty, but as an insurance against the consequences of their sexual choices. They elected therefore to undergo testing more or less frequently, on the basis of their knowledge of their sexual activity at a given time. They had numerous tests in some periods, and no tests in other periods, a behaviour which was not a very efficient preventive strategy, to put it mildly.

The women of the *favela* studied by Gregg equated health risk with not having a Pap smear. Women who failed to do *prevençao* were seen as lazy and irresponsible. The general belief that diligent employment of the Pap test would protect women from sexually transmitted infections led to a neglect of other safety measures, such as the use of condoms or verification of their sexual partner as a carrier of a venereal disease. The creative use of the Pap test by women in the *favela* as an insurance against dangers of sexuality, Jessica Gregg explains, gave them some behavioural elbow room. Unfortunately, it also severely limited the benefits of screening for cervical malignancies, and opened the way to patterns of sexual behaviour that put their health at risk.

Women from the *favela* who did develop cervical cancer usually blamed themselves, and sometimes also other women, but hardly ever men or the conditions in which they lived. The reinterpretation of cervical cancer as a sexually transmitted pathology firmly linked it with women's inappropriate sexual behaviour. This disease combined the stigma of cancer (still seen as 'catching' in the popular imagination) with that of venereal disease. Even a woman who remained faithful to her husband attributed her disease to the fact that she continued to desire her husband, in spite of the fact that he may have left her temporarily for another woman. Her frustration, and her excessive and 'unhealthy' sexual drive, produced a cancer. Women who had chosen 'liberty' viewed cervical cancer as a direct consequence of this choice. Cancer became linked with sexual impurity, and its treatment was equated with purification through the abandonment of all sexual activity. Some women underwent hysterectomy, an operation which, many of them believed, made them asexual. Other women underwent radiation therapy, a treatment which often induces the narrowing and thinning of the vagina (vaginal stenosis). This latter condition can make sexual intercourse painful or even impossible. Cancer patients interviewed by Jessica Gregg frequently reported that they had lost the pleasure of sex. They saw this, however, as a positive development. Elimination of the source of their deviant behaviour erased their sin and made a new start in life possible. As one cancer patient explained: 'I'm like virgin again; its like I'm fifteen'.[14]

Purification, cure, and a new beginning could have provided a happy ending to stories of women with cervical cancer. Alas, the great majority of the *favela* women were diagnosed with advanced tumours. Cancer treatment is fully covered by the Brazilian national health service SUS, and all the women studied by Jessica Gregg received free treatment in the local public hospital. On the other hand, they received standardized radiation therapy (an individualized treatment was reserved to patients with a private health insurance), sometimes had to wait a long time for a free hospital bed, were left to their own devices to cope with the harsh secondary effects of their treatment, and were rarely cured. Their chances of cure, often not very high anyway, were often further compromised by difficulty in completing all the prescribed radiation sessions (sometimes because they did not have money for a bus fare) and their poor general health. In spite of the considerable investment in the development of *prevençao* in Recife and the dedication of health professionals who implemented the screening programmes, Jessica Gregg's narrative helps us understand why these well-intentioned efforts were not translated into an important decrease in mortality from cervical cancer.

HPV vaccine: not for those who need it most?

All the experts agree that an HPV vaccine, if efficient, will be highly beneficial for developing countries. In industrialized countries the HPV vaccine is expected to further reduce the already low incidence of cervical malignancies and to reduce iatrogenic effects of screening for this disease. In developing countries, especially those with a high frequency of cervical cancer, the main problem is not how to perfect health services and provide women with a maximal level of protection, but how to reduce the unacceptably high level of mortality from this disease.

Public health experts constructed mathematical models that attempted to find out how to best use limited resources and provide an optimal—and least expensive—combination of vaccination and screening, which would lead to the largest possible reduction in the frequency of cervical cancers. They also discussed the role of cultural factors, such as religious barriers, cultural taboos, and misconceptions, that may influence the HPV vaccine's acceptability. Misconceptions, coupled with generalized suspicion of Western medicine, may play an especially dangerous role. A vaccine destined for girls and associated with a sexually transmitted infection may exacerbate rumours, such as the vaccine being a plot to sterilize young girls. Experts have therefore stressed the need for educating local population and producing a receptive environment for efficient vaccination. For now, however, all these debates deal with a non-existent problem. In the early twenty-first century the main obstacle to the use of of an HPV vaccine outside industrialized countries is not cultural obstacles but its price. No developing or middle-range country can conceive a mass vaccination campaign in which the protection of each woman costs several hundred dollars.

The producers of the HPV vaccines have promised to make it accessible to developing countries. Nevertheless, during the first 4 years of marketing such vaccines the companies have focused exclusively on sales in industrialized countries. This may change in the future, especially if the developing countries themselves, international bodies, and non-governmental organizations exert pressure on manufacturers of the vaccine for HPV. A demonstration that the HPV vaccine prevents invasive cervical tumours and not only the iatrogenic effects of screening for these tumours may spur such pressures. Alternatively, middle-income countries with important pharmaceutical industries and a solid scientific infrastructure, such as India, Thailand, China, Brazil, or South Korea, may take over the mass production of an inexpensive HPV vaccine, either through an agreement with the patent holders, a contestation of the patents in the name of the public good, or a combination of these two strategies. Both solutions—the agreement of the producers of the existing HPV vaccines to drastically lower their prices in non-industrialized countries, and the rise of 'South–South' networks of manufacture and distribution of a cheaper HPV vaccine—are plausible, and either or both may follow a demonstration of the capacity of this vaccine to prevent cancer in developing countries. In the meantime, all the discussions on vaccination against HPV outside Western countries remain theoretical. As this book went to press the HPV vaccine was still a rich person's luxury and could be afforded only by women who have a relatively low risk of developing a cervical malignacy.

An infectious, sexually transmitted cancer in context

Cervical cancer, public health experts and propaganda leaflets repeat, is a 'fully preventable disease'. There is, however, a big difference between preventability—a hypothetical variable—and the construction of efficient preventive programmes. In the twentieth century medical sciences devised efficient ways to reduce the number of women who suffer from advanced cervical malignancies. The persistence of the disease in many parts of the world reflects to an important extent a failure to act upon economic and social conditions that hamper the diffusion of preventive measures. In the first half of the twentieth century, directors of the Rockefeller Foundation believed that the reduction of disease burden in developing countries would lead to a quasi-automatic improvement of the economic situation of people who live in these countries. In 1951, the former director of the Rockefeller Foundation Wilbur Sawyer was obliged to recognize that poor health is usually the consequence of poverty, not the other way round: 'the problem is much broader than health, which cannot flourish in an adverse socio-economic environment'.[15]

In the first half of the twentieth century, the prevalent image of malignant tumours was one of a pathology linked with urbanization and technological progress. 'Primitive people', researchers argued, rarely suffered from malignancies. When these people migrated to industrialized countries and adopted the lifestyle of more affluent societies their rates of cancer rose sharply. Cancer was rare among Africans who lived in Africa, but became much more frequent among African Americans, especially those who lived in the cities. The view of cancer as a disease of civilization, and, for some, the price human beings were paying for the abandonment of a simpler and healthier lifestyle, became more difficult to sustain when researchers started to look for links between affluence and specific malignancies. They had found that some cancers, such as breast cancer, are more frequent in women of higher socio-economic status (although they have worse outcomes in poor women). Other cancers, such as head and neck tumours and cervical cancer, are associated with a lower socio-economic status. Others still, such as lung cancer, were once seen as independent of income (men of all social strata smoked) but then became associated with low income and low status.

In the early twentieth century epidemiologists uncovered the correlation between poverty and cervical cancer. Working-class women, and those in low-income brackets, have the highest incidence of this disease. In the early twenty-first century this is still true within each given society, but the most dramatic division is the one that separates poor and affluent countries. In some of the poorest regions of the Earth cervical cancer continues to be the leading cause of cancer death among women. Some middle-income countries, especially in Latin America and South-east Asia, also have relatively high levels of cervical tumours. Many among the latter countries implemented nationwide programmes of screening for this disease. The success of these programmes is, we have seen, uneven. Nevertheless it is reasonable to assume that middle-income countries will be able to reduce the occurrence of cervical malignancies, although it is not certain what the pace and the extent of such a reduction will be.

The situation in poor developing countries is very different. When funds available for health care are severely limited, specialists and politicians tend to concentrate above all on diseases that kill children, such as diarrhoea, pneumonia, measles, malaria, and tetanus, not on those that affect middle-aged people. Prevention of childhood diseases is relatively inexpensive, can be made without important investments in health infrastructure, and is especially efficient in terms of gaining years of productive life. Public health experts in developing countries are aware of the suffering produced by cervical cancer, but when resources are rare they are obliged to make difficult choices. Such choices become even more drastic in a period of slow economic growth and decreasing investment in international aid. Barring proof of the high efficacy of the HPV vaccine coupled with a precipitous drop in its price, it is difficult to be optimistic about a rapid reduction in the occurrence of cervical cancer in low-income countries.

EPILOGUE:
CERVICAL CANCER IN THE
TWENTY-FIRST CENTURY

I n autumn 2003 my graduate student, Nina H., wrote to tell me that she had been diagnosed with cervical cancer. Nina, a Mexican, studied biology at the Autonomous University of Mexico, worked a few years as editor for a scientific journal, then entered a graduate programme on the history of science in Paris. She was very bright, intellectually curious, hardworking, vivacious, funny, and warm. In the final stages of her PhD she went back to Mexico City to finish writing her thesis, an endeavour somewhat slowed down by the birth of her second child. Her diagnosis was totally unexpected. Nina had no known risk factors for cervical cancer and no previous warnings. She diligently underwent periodic Pap smears, all of which were normal. The news about her cancer was distressing, but Nina and her family were hopeful, and so was I. She had access to good-quality medical care and her doctors had told her that her cancer was found at an early stage, and she had very good chances of being cured. Nina underwent a hysterectomy and radiotherapy, recovered rapidly, and went back to the writing of her thesis. Alas, a few months later she developed back and abdominal pain and was diagnosed with disseminated cancer.

All attempts to halt the rapid progress of her tumour failed. Nina died in spring 2004; she was 34 years old.

Nina was very unlucky. Regular Pap smears are an efficient way of preventing cervical malignancies and tumours limited to the cervix are often cured. Unfortunately, the Pap smear is not a one-hundred-percent sure diagnostic method. Cytologists make mistakes, some results are false negative, and rapidly growing cancers cannot be detected by regular screening. Moreover, in some cases a malignant tumour which seems to be small and localized has already produced invisible distant metastases at the time it is diagnosed. The proposal that cervical cancer is a 'preventable disease' does not mean that it can be always prevented. Women who 'do everything right' can still die from a cervical malignancy.

An aggressive and incurable malignancy is always very distressing, but at least Nina passed away quietly at her home, with her family beside her. 'Annie', a 67-year-old British woman described by the anthropologist Julia Lawson, was even less lucky. Annie was diagnosed with a cervical cancer, underwent a hysterectomy and postoperative radiotherapy, and was believed to be cured. A year later her doctors found that she was suffering from a generalized, incurable cancer. Annie's health deteriorated rapidly, and she expressed her wish to die in her home. When she developed a recto-vaginal fistula and became incontinent, Annie changed her mind however, and asked to be admitted to a hospice, mainly because she did not wish her family to witness her bodily degradation. Placed in a common ward, Annie was perceived as a nuisance by other patients, greatly distressed by her smell. The hospice workers faced a very difficult choice: either to put Annie in an isolated room and to make the final period of her life miserable, or to keep her in contact with other patients, and to make their last days more difficult . They elected an intermediate solution: Annie was left in the common ward, but when other beds on the ward became empty they were not filled by other patients. As her disease progressed, Annie, increasingly depressed by her condition, asked to be sedated; she was then moved to an isolated room. She died while sedated.[1]

Annie's story displays ruptures and continuities in the treatment of cervical cancer over the last 200 years. When Annie was diagnosed with cervical cancer she was treated promptly with a hysterectomy and radiotherapy, and her doctors had hoped that she was cured. At that point, her fate looked very different from that of women diagnosed with cancer of the womb in the nineteenth century. However, when a year later Annie's doctors discovered that her cancer had spread, they were nearly as powerless as the physicians who took care of women with uterine tumours a century and a half earlier. Like their predecessors, the only treatment they were able to offer their patient was painkillers and sedatives.

In industrialized countries, stories such as those of Nina and Annie have become increasingly rare. In the nineteenth and early twentieth centuries, cancer of the womb was a frequent and very scary disease. It was sometimes a shorthand for the horrors of cancer, as in a dialogue from the second act of Alban Berg's opera, *Woyzeck* (composed between 1914 and 1922):

> Doctor: A woman died, in four weeks! Carcinoma uteri. I already had twenty patients with this disease. In four weeks....
>
> Captain: Doctor, please don't scare me. There are people who died from fear, from pure fear.

Doctor: In four weeks! It will be an interesting autopsy.
Captain: Oh, oh, oh![2]

One may assume that, the mention of 'carcinoma uteri' in present-day Germany or Austria will not produce shrieks of fear. In Europe and North America, the relative rarity of this disease has partly obliterated its earlier terrifying images. In the twenty-first century fear of cancer has shifted to other malignant tumours; for women, above all, breast cancer. The disappearance of the image of cervical cancer as an iconic dread disease should not be confused, however, with the disappearance of cervical cancer. For many women in Asia, Africa, and Latin America, cervical cancer is not a remote risk but an omnipresent danger.

Writing about AIDS in 1990, the cultural studies scholar Paula Treichler coined the term 'epidemic of signification'. This term points to the dense tangle of significations of a deadly, transmissible disease, linked with sex and the use of illegal drugs, and which selectively killed male homosexuals and inner-city dwellers. Twenty years later, AIDS continues to be linked to sex among men, drugs, and the trade in sexual services. The main meaning of this epidemic, however, has shifted to the deadly effects of poverty and under-development, especially (but not exclusively) in sub-Saharan Africa. Cervical cancer has undergone a similar transformation.

For poor women in Recife, Brazil, at high risk of this disease, 'cervical cancer was almost absurdly loaded with metaphoric potential'.[3] This disease continues to be linked with women's reproductive organs, the risks of female (but not male) sexual behaviour, contamination and decay, purity, and danger. However, in the early twenty-first century the main meaning of this pathology is the disproportional plight of poor women in developing countries. Cervical cancer is, like AIDS, a demonstrative pathology. It demonstrates the possibility of reducing the cancer burden thanks to scientific progress, but also the limitations of purely technological solutions to health problems. It makes visible social inequalities, discrimination against women, the dramatic consequences of instable, disrupted, and chaotic lives, and the contrasting ways in which biomedical knowledge changes lives in affluent and resource-poor societies.

In 1967 the Brazilian hygienist Adonis de Carvalho noted that because cervical tumours are especially frequent in the north of Brazil, some doctors classified this pathology as a tropical disease. This is, de Carvalho proposed, a misleading view. The high frequency of cervical tumours in northern Brazil is not related to climate, but reflects a combination of malnutrition, poor hygiene, early sexual maturation, lack of medical services, and an elevated number of pregnancies. Less-affluent regions of Western countries also have higher rates of cervical cancer than the more affluent ones. 'Tropical', de Carvalho concluded, 'frequently stands for poor.' The equation of cervical tumours with poverty is also true today. The majority of premature deaths from cervical malignancies worldwide are, as de Carvalho put it, 'a drama of misery, ignorance and social suffering'.[4] Women who live in poorer parts of the world are frequently as disarmed when facing cervical cancer now as were European and North American women a century and half ago. The first few chapters of this book are not only a description of a long-forgotten past.

GLOSSARY

ASCUS (atypical squamous cells of unknown significance) Unusual-looking cells found in a vaginal smear (i.e. the Pap smear) that cannot be clearly classified as precancerous.

BRACHYTHERAPY Treatment by radiation source (such as radium) placed in the immediate vicinity of the target. In oncology, the radiation source, usually in thin glass or metal tubes (called radium needles) or glass spheres (radium seeds), is placed near the targeted tumour.

BIOPSY The analysis of excised tissue that is fixed, stained, and observed under a microscope. Biopsy can be excisional, the removal of a whole suspicious area (as is often the case when analysing a lump, mole, or wart), or incisional, when only a sample of tissue is removed.

CARCINOMA IN SITU (intraepithelial neoplasia) A lesion composed of cells which look exactly like cancer cells, but which do not invade other tissues.

CAUTERIZATION Elimination of diseases tissues by 'burning' them with a hot iron, corrosive chemical substances, or a galvanic current.

CERVIX The uterine cervix or the neck of the uterus; the narrow, lower part of the uterus, which joins the upper part of the vagina.

CHEMOTHERAPY When used in the context of cancer therapy, chemotherapy refers to treatment with drugs which selectively destroy rapidly multiplying cells, and, for this reason, harm more malignant cells than normal cells.

COLPOSCOPY A diagnostic procedure during which the cervix and the vagina are observed with a special instrument, the colposcope, a specially adapted variant of the binocular microscope. If suspicious areas are identified, the physician performing the examination (the colposcopist) will often take biopsies (tissue samples) from these areas.

CORPUS UTERI The uterine body; the upper, larger part of the uterus, linked to the cervix.

CURETTAGE The scraping of diseased or suspected tissues with a sharp instrument, to either eliminate them or facilitate microscopic diagnosis.

DYSPLASIA The abnormal proliferation of cells.

ENDOMETRIUM Tissue that lines the interior of the uterine cavity. Cancer of the endometrium is the more recent name for cancer of the uterine body.

FIBROID A benign tumour of the uterus.

FISTULA An abnormal connection between two organs or vessels. The destruction of tissues by progressing cervical cancer can produce an abnormal connection between the vagina and the urethra or between the vagina and the anus and permanent leaks of urine or faeces. Also, a fistula can be a complication of cancer radiotherapy, or of surgery for this disease.

HAEMORRHAGE A massive loss of blood.

HIV (human immunodeficiency virus) The virus which causes AIDS.

HPV (human papilloma virus) A sexually transmitted human virus. Some HPV strains cause genital warts; others increase the probability of developing cervical cancer. HPV is also linked to some head and neck tumours. HPV is highly infectious, and the majority of sexually active people acquire this virus; but only a minority remain permanently infected with a 'dangerous' strain.

HYSTERECTOMY Surgical ablation of the uterus. Surgery may be radical (removal of the uterus and surrounding tissues), total (removal of the whole uterus), or subtotal (leaving the cervix intact). The latter surgery is never done for cancer.

IATROGENIC DISEASE A disease or distressing symptom induced by medical intervention, either by mistake (e.g. accidental infection acquired in a hospital) or because the therapy had important side effects (e.g. burns produced by radiotherapy of cancer).

MASTECTOMY Surgical ablation of the breast.

OVARIECTOMY Surgical ablation of the ovaries.

PALLIATIVE TREATMENT Treatment that is undergone not to cure a disease, only to alleviate its distressing symptoms.

PAP SMEAR (*also known as* Papanicolaou test, cervical smear, exfoliative cytology) A test that detects precancerous lesions of the cervix. After the application of a speculum, a tool—usually a wooden spatula—is used to gather a sample of cells from the cervix. The cells are then stained and examined under a microscope.

RADIOTHERAPY Elimination of malignant cells by radiation; this may be X-rays, or radiation produced by a radioactive element such as radium. The latter approach, called radiation therapy, can be made through implantation of radioactive seeds or needles in the proximity of the tumour, or from a distance, using a more powerful source of radiation.

RECURRENCE Return of a malignant tumour after its elimination through surgery, radiotherapy, chemotherapy, or a combination of these approaches.

SCIRRHOUS A nineteenth-century term describing indurations or tumefaction of tissues which could become a 'true' cancer.

SEE-AND-TREAT METHOD Elimination of visually identified cervical lesions with cryotherapy (destruction of cells by cold, using products such as liquid nitrogen) without attempting to make a more precise, microscopic diagnosis of the nature of the treated lesion.

SEPSIS A generalized infection.

SPECULUM A medical tool used to examine body cavities. The most common is the vaginal speculum, employed to examine the vagina and the cervix, to take tissue and cell samples, and to apply medication. The vaginal speculum is usually a hollow cylinder with a rounded end that is divided into two hinged parts. It can be made from either steel (to be reused) or plastic (for a single use). The speculum is inserted into the vagina to dilate it and make it accessible to the examiner's gaze.

Teletherapy Radiation therapy, in which a powerful radiation source (such as a radium 'bomb', a large quantity of radium) is placed at distance from the target (usually a malignant tumour).

VIA method (visual inspection with acetic acid) Direct examination of the cervix after application of dilute (5%) acetic acid. Zones of abnormal cell proliferation appear as white spots or patches. This method is proposed as a cheaper and simpler way to screen for cervical cancer in developing countries, because there is no need for an expert reading of microscopic preparations in a laboratory, and the visual examination can be performed by any trained health worker.

NOTES

Prologue

1. Bette A. Toole, *Ada, The Enchantress of Numbers: A Selection of Letters*, Mill Valley, CA: Strawberry Press, 1992. Lovelace's letter to her mother, early 1852 (p. 412); Lovelace's letter to her mother, 12 July 1852 (p. 418).

2. Toole, *Ada, The Enchantress of Numbers*. Lovelace's letter to her mother, early August 1852 (p. 420).

3. Nelson Castro, *Los ultimos dias de Eva: Historia de un engano*, Buenos Aires: Vergara Editor, 2007. This book is based on Ivanissevich's testimony. Ivanissevich's version, such as reported by Castro, is puzzling. The symptoms of a cervical tumour are different from those of appendicitis, and if indeed uterine malignancy was suspected it is not clear why Péron's doctors waited for more than 20 months to perform a gynaecological examination.

4. Castro, *Los ultimos dias de Eva*, annexe 2, p. 132.

5. Lawrence Altman, 'From the life of Evita, a new chapter on medical secrecy', *New York Times*, 6 June 2000.

6. This detail is mentioned in a memoir written by Eva Péron's doctor, Jorge Albertelli, more than 40 years after the events. Jorge Albertelli, *Las 'Cien dias' de Eva Peron*, Buenos Aires: Cesarini Hermanos Editores, 1994.

7. Such rumours were reported in Nicholas Faser's and Marysa Navarro's book, *Eva Péron*, New York: WW Norton & Company, 1980. Born in an atmosphere of intense palace intrigue, rumours that shed negative light on Juan Péron might have been inaccurate.

8. Information about Goody's life and illness was mainly gathered from press articles: James Sturcke, 'Cancer tests go up after Goody diagnosis', *The Guardian*, 17 February 2009; Carol Midgley, 'Jade Goody: why resent the brutal reality show that her dying has become?', *The Times*, 19 February 2009; Sarah Lyall, 'Jade Goody, British reality TV star, dies', *New York Times*, 23 March 2009; Jenny Percival, 'Jade Goody dies of cancer', *The Guardian*, 22 March 2009; Sarah Boseley, 'Jade Goody: celebrity's fatal illness changed cervical cancer attitudes', *The Guardian*, 22 March 2009; Peter Beresford, 'The hidden side of death', *The Guardian*, 12 March 2009; Madeleine Bunting, 'In bewildering times, Jade's story of sacrifice offers us the ultimate reality', *The Guardian*, 9 March 2009.

9. Jeremy Laurance, 'Charity calls for lowering of age for first smear tests', *The Independent*, 17 February 2009; Jenny Hope, 'Defeat for Jade Goody campaign as cervical cancer screening age will NOT be lowered in England', *Daily Mail*, 25 June 2009.

10. Jade Goody, 'I ignored cancer warnings', *Heat*, 27 August 2008, http://sify.com/movies/fullstory.php?id=14747451.

Chapter 1

1. Quoted by Henry Sigerist, 'The historical development of pathology and therapy of cancer', *Bulletin of the New York Academy of Medicine*, 1939: 642–653, on p. 648.

2. W.P. Baldwin, quoted in James Marion Sims, *The Story of My Life*, New York: Appleton, 1884, p. 434.

3. Jean Paul Mayre, *Quelques considérations sur le squirrhe et le cancer en général et du squirrhe de l'utérus en particulier*, Paris: Imprimerie Didot le Jeune, 1823, p. 11.

4. J.A.H. Marie Auguste Rossignol, *Essai sur le cancer de l'utérus*, Montpellier: Coucourdan Imprimeur, 1806, p. 11.

5. Robert Barnes, *A Clinical History of Medical and Surgical Diseases of Women*, London: J&A Churchill, 1878, p. 821.

6. Edmund Rigby, *Constitutional Treatment of Female Diseases*, London: Henry Renshaw, 1857, p. 214.

7. Rossignol, *Essai sur le cancer de l'utérus*, p. 10.

8. Pierre Jerome Sebastien Téallier, *Du cancer de la matrice, de ses causes, son diagnostic et son traitement*, Paris: Ballière, 1836, p. 108.

9. Charles D. Meigs, *Woman: Her Diseases and Remedies*, 4th edn, Philadelphia: Blanchard & Lea, 1859, p. 333.

10. Joseph Claude Anthelme Récamier, *Recherches sur le traitement de cancer*, Paris: Gabon, 1829, tome 1, p. 317.

11. Bernard Lejeune, *Traitement du cancer du col de l'utérus par la cautérisation au chlorure du zinc*, Paris: A. Prent Imprimeur, 1879, pp. 34–37.

12. William Goodell, *Lessons in Gynecology*, Philadelphia: D. Brinton, 1880, p. 234. The Goodell pouch is the extension of the peritoneal cavity between the rectum and the back wall of the uterus.

13. Rossignol, *Essai sur le cancer de l'utérus*, p. 6.

14. Narcisse Desiré Mury, *Du cancer de l'utérus et de sa thérapeutique*, Paris: Imprimerie Didot le Jeune, 1826, p. 9.

15. Paul Broca, *Traité des tumeurs*, vol. 1, Paris: J.B. Ballière, 1866, p. 590.

Chapter 2

1. E.T. Thring, 'On the radical abdominal operation for uterine cancer', *Journal of Obstetrics and Gynaecology*, 1907, pp. 239–245, on p. 245.

2. L. Goustave Richelot, *L'hystérectomie vaginale contre le cancer d'utérus et les affectation non cancéreuses*, Paris: Goustave Doin, 1894, p. 45.

3. Charles P. Noble, 'Early diagnosis and operation in cancer of the uterus', *American Gynecological Journal* (Toledo, OH), December, 1892, in: *Collection of Gynecological Reprints*, Countway Medicine Rare Books, 24.D.84, no. 19.

4. Joseph M. Baldy, 'Carcinoma of the uterus', *Proceedings of the Medical Society of the State of Pennsylvania*, May 1883, in: Countway Medicine Rare Books, 24.D.84, no. 2.

5. Samuel Pozzi, *A Treatise on Gynaecology, Clinical and Operative*, vol. 2, London: The New Syndham Society, 1893, p. 57.

6. Joseph Bouvier, *De l'état actuel la thérapeutique radicale du cancer de l'utérus*, Lyon: Imprimerie Schneider, 1904, p. 67.

7. Edwin Ricketts, 'Early diagnosis of cancer of the uterus', paper presented to the *Cincinnati Obstetrical Society*, 14 June 1895.

8. Frederich Winckel, *A Handbook of Diseases of Women*, Edinburgh and London: Young J. Petland, 1890, p. 367.

9. Alfred Duhrssen, *A Manual of Gynecological Practice*, London: H.K. Lewis, 1985, p. 190.

10. A.N.L. Lewers, *Cancer of the Uterus*, Philadelpia: P. Blackiston's Sons & Co., 1902, p. v.

11. Mary A. Dixon Jones, 'Colpo-hysterectomy for malignant disease', *American Journal of Obstetrics and Diseases of Women and Children*, 1893, vol. 27(4–5), in: Countway Medicine Rare Books, 24.D.80, no. 19.

12. Regina Morantz-Sanchez, 'Negotiating power at the bedside: historical perspectives on nineteenth-century patients and their gynaecologists', *Feminist Studies*, 2000, 26(2): 287–309, on p. 301.

13. Louisa Garrett Anderson and Kate Platt, 'Malignant disease of the uterus: a digest of 265 cases treated in the New Hospital for Women', *Obstetrics and Gynaecology of the British Empire*, 1908, 14(6): 381–392.

Chapter 3

1. Barton Cooke Hirst, *A Text-book of Diseases of Women*, Philadelphia: W.B. Saunders & Co, 1903, p. 261.

2. Richard J. Cowen, *X-rays: Their Employment in Cancer and Other Diseases*, London: Henry J. Glaisher, 1904, p. 83.

3. Daniel Thomas Quigley, *The Conquest of Cancer by Radium and Other Methods*, Philadelphia: F.A. Davis Company, 1929, p. xi.

4. Janet E. Lane-Claypon, *Cancer of the Uterus: A Statistical Inquiry Into the Results of Treatment, Being an Analysis of the Existing Literature,*

Reports on Public Health and Medical Subjects, no. 40, London: Ministry of Health, 1927, p. v.

5. Vita Sackville-West, *The Marie Curie Hospital*, 1947, p. 20, quoted in: Ornella Moscucci, 'The ineffable masonry of sex: feminist surgeons and the establishement of radiotherapy in early twentieth century Britain', *Bulletin of the History of Medicine*, 2007, 81: 139–163, on p. 158.

6. Quoted by Rene Hugenin, 'L'apport de la France à l'étude du cancer', in A. Théophile Alajouanine *et al.*, *Ce que la France a apporté à la médicine*, Paris: Flammarion, 1946, pp. 141–172, on p. 166.

7. Barbara Clow, 'Who is afraid of Susan Sontag? Or the myths and metaphors of cancer reconsidered', *Social History of Medicine*, 2001, 14(2): 293–312, on p. 301.

8. Patients' records 1920–1940, Archive Department, Curie Institute, Paris.

9. Elisabeth Hurdon, *Cancer of the Uterus*, Oxford: Oxford University Press, 1942, p. 112.

10. Letter of Dr Edward Skinner, from Kansas City, 16 March 1937, Columbia University Health Sciences Library, Archives and Special Collections, Maurice Lenz Papers, Box 12, file 1. Correspondence relating to the survey of the standardization committee of the American Radium society concerning treatment of cancer of the uterine cervix.

11. Franz Buschke, Simeon T. Cantril, and Herbert M. Parker, *Supervoltage Roenetgenotherapy*, Springfield, IL: Charles Thomas, 1950, p. 239.

12. Hurdon, *Cancer of the Uterus*, p. 112.

13. Patients' records 1920–1940. Archive Department, Curie Institute, Paris.

14. Nigel Paneth, Ezra Susser, and Mervyn Susser, 'Origins and early development of case control study. Part 2, The case control study from Lane-Claypon to 1950', *Sozial und Preventivemedizin*, 2002, 47: 359–365.

15. Janet E. Lane-Claypon, *A Report on the Treatment of Cancer of the Uterus at the Samaritan Free Hospital*, Reports on Public Health and Medical Subjects, no. 47, London: Ministry of Health, 1927, p. 33.

16. Lane-Claypon, *A Report on the Treatment of Cancer of the Uterus*, p. 7.

17. Editorial, 'Results of treatment of uterine cancer', *British Medical Journal*, 14 January, 1928, i: 69.

18. Robert Duval and Antoine Lacasagne, *Classification pratique des cancers derivés des epithelium cutanés and cutaneo-muceux*, Paris: Octave Doin, 1922, p. 6.

19. Note of C. Regaud, 'Erreurs a rectifier dans les listes du Dr. Lacasagne' [mistakes to be rectified in Dr. Lacasagne's list], joined to the typed notes: *Cervical Cancer, 1930s*, Box 'Gynecological cancers', Archive Department, Curie Institute, Paris.

Chapter 4

1. R. Francis Matters, *The Cervix Uteri, With Specific Reference to the Development of Cancer*, Adelaide: The Hassel Press, 1935, p. 155.

2. Walter Schiller, 'Clinical behaviour of early carcinoma of the cervix', *Surgery, Gynecology and Obstetrics*, 1938, 66(2): 129–140, on p. 138.

3. Mr Duran, 'The campaign against cancer', *Journal of the National Medical Association*, 1946, 38(1): 24–26, on p. 25.

4. Catherine Macfarlane, Margaret C. Sturgis, and Faith Fetterman, 'Periodic examination of the female pelvic organs and breasts: a report of a fifteen years research on the control of cancer', *CA Cancer Journal for Clinicians*, 1953, 3: 205–207, on p. 205.

5. George N. Papanicolaou and Herbert F. Traut, 'The diagnostic value of vaginal smears in carcinoma of the uterus', *American Journal of Obstetrics and Gynecology*, 1941, 42: 193–206, on pp. 193–194.

6. Bayard Carter, Kenneth Cuyler, Walter L. Thomas, Robert Creadick, and Robert Alter, 'The methods of managment of

carcinoma in situ of the cervix', *American Journal of Obstetrics and Gynecology*, 1952, 64: 833–845.

7. John E. Dunn, 'The relationships between carcinoma in situ and invasive cervical carcinoma: a consideration of the contribution to the problem to be made from general population data', *Cancer*, 1953, 6(5): 873–886. At that time the definition of dysplasia varied greatly, making precise evaluations difficult.

8. Edward E. Sieler, 'Microdiagnosis of carcinoma in situ of the uterine cervix', *Cancer*, 1956, 9(3): 463–469.

9. Olaf Petersen, *Precancerous Changes of the Cervical Epithelium*, Acta Radiologica, supplement 127, Copenhagen: Danish Science Press, 1955.

10. Leopold G. Koss, Frederick Stewart, Frank Foote *et al.*, 'Some histological aspects of behaviour of epidermoid carcinoma in situ and related lesions of uterine cervix. A long term prospective study', *Cancer*, 1963, 12: 1160–1211.

11. Papers of the Arthur Purdy Stout Society of surgical pathologists. Box 1, papers 1957–1986, folder 6. Undated, probably 1970s. Columbia University Health Sciences Library, Archives and Special Collections.

12. Linda Bryder, *Women, Bodies and Medical Science: An Inquiry Into Cervical Cancer*, Basingstoke: Palgrave Macmillan, 2010.

13. Joanna Manning (ed.), *The Cartwright Papers Essays on the Cervical Cancer Inquiry of 1987–88*, Auckland: Bridget Williams Books, 2010.

14. More recently, the introduction of tests for infection with 'dangerous' strains of human papilloma virus (HPV; discussed in Chapter 6) helps to resolve some of the uncertainties of ASCUS diagnosis, although it does not eliminate them totally.

15. Lisa Spinelli, 'Living with HPV', *Boston Phonenix*, 4 September 2009.

16. Vered Levy-Barzilai, 'Hey doc! It hurts', *Haaretz*, English edition, 14 February, 2006.

17. Anette Forss, Carol Tishelman, Catarina Widmark, and Lisbeth Sachs, 'Women's experiences of cervical cellular changes: an

unintentional transition from health to liminality?', *Sociology of Health & Illness*, 2004, 26(3): 306–325, on p. 317.

18. Anette Forss *et al.*, 'Women's experiences of cervical cellular changes', p. 317.

19. Nicky Britten, 'Personal view: colposcopy', *British Medical Journal*, 1988, i: 296.

20. Shanon Brownlee, *Overtreated: Why So Much Medicine is Making Us Sicker and Poorer*, New York: Bloomsbury, 2008, p. 203.

Chapter 5

1. Julien Bertre, *Essai sur le cancer de l'utérus*, Paris: Imprimerie Didot le Jeune, 1824, p. 29.

2. Anstruth Milligan, 'The crusade against cancer of the uterus', *Journal of Obstetrics and Gynaecology*, 1907, 11: 45–63, on p. 58.

3. Milligan, p. 62.

4. Maurice B. Judd, 'Art aids the doctor', *Hygiea*, 17 (February 1939), reproduced in: Leslie Reagan, 'Engendering the dread disease', *American Journal of Public Health*, 1997, 87(11): 1179–1187.

5. Advice for medical lecturers who speak to lay public, leaflet, 1936, box 90, BECC papers, Wellcome Library.

6. Quoted in Kirsten Gardner, *Early Detection: Women, Cancer and Awarness in the Twentieth Century*, Chapel Hill, NC: University of North Carolina, 2006, p. 45.

7. Catherine Macfarlane, Margaret C. Sturgis, and Faith Fetterman, 'Periodic examination of the female pelvic organs and breasts: a report of a fifteen years research on the control of cancer', *CA Cancer Journal for Clinicians*, 1953, 3: 205–207, on p. 205.

8. Germaine Lavignac, 'La Lutte anti-cancereuse aux Etats-Unis', *La Lutte Contre le Cancer*, 1928, 5(19): 139–150.

9. Annual report of the Curie Foundation for 1932. Minutes of meeting of the foundations' administration council of 4 May 1934. Archive of the Curie Institute, Paris.

10. Simone Laborde, 'Le cancer de l'utérus et sa prevention', *ACTA de l'Union internationale contre le cancer*, 1937, 2(3): 244–255, on p. 250.

11. Walter Schiller, 'Early diagnosis of carcinoma of the cervix', *Surgery, Gynecology and Obstetrics*, 1933, 56: 212–222, on p. 220.

12. 'Advancement of science', *Time*, 11 January 1937.

13. Catherine Macfarlane papers. Medical College of Philadelphia archive, account 47, Box 2, Folder 23, typed manuscript, 'The inside history of the periodic pelvic examination research'. Quoted by Robert Aronowitz, 'Gardasil: a vaccine against cancer and a drug to reduce risk', paper presented at the conference Cancer Vaccines for Girls, Rutgers University, 26–27 September 2008.

14. Catherine Macfarlane *et al.* 'Periodic examination of the female pelvic organs and breasts: a report of a fifteen years research on the control of cancer', p. 205.

15. Howard C. Taylor, 'Controversial points in the treatment of carcinoma of the cervix', *Cancer*, 1952, 5: 435–441, on p. 437.

16. Malcolm Donaldson, 'Education of the public concerning cancer', Medical Officer, 9 September 1950, box 90, BECC papers, Wellcome Library, Archives and Manuscripts Department, series SA/CRC. The ACS, this test attests, was especially active in promoting diagnoses of 'precancerous conditions'.

17. Wellcome Library, Archives and Manuscripts Department, series SA/MWF, Documents of the Medical Women's Federation, file F.13/3.

18. Preliminary debates on cervical cancer screening, House of Lords, vol. 269, no. 120, 2 November 1965. Documents of the Medical Women's Federation, file F.13/3.

19. Talk by John Wakefield, Head of Department of Social Research, Christie Hospital and Holt Radium Institute, and Chairman of the Committee on Public Education of International Union Against Cancer, 27 March 1968. Documents of the Medical Women's Federation, file F. 13/5.

20. Women's National Cancer Control Campaign (previously National Cervical Cancer Prevention Campaign), Report on Activities, 1968. Documents of the Medical Women's Federation, file F. 13/5.

21. World Health Organization, *Comprehensive Cervical Cancer Control: A Guide to Essential Practice*, Geneva: World Health Organization, 2006. www.who.int/reproductivehealth/publications/cancers/9241547006/en/index.html.

22. Jerome Groopman, 'Health care: who knows best', *New York Review of Books*, 11 February 2010.

23. Andran A. Renshaw, 'Editorial. Increased cervical cancer risk screening intervals: a risky investment,' *Diagnostic Cytology*, 2004, 30(3): 137–138.

24. This problem was discussed in 1999 during US Congress debates on screening for cervical and breast cancers. Hearings before the Sub-Committee on Health and Environment of the Committee on Commerce, House of Representatives, One Hundred Sixth Congress, 21 July 1999, Washington DC: US Government Printing Office, 1999.

25. http://info.cancerresearchuk.org/cancerstats/mortality/.

26. Julian Peto, Clare Gilham, Olivia Fletcher, and Fiona E. Matthews, 'The cervical cancer epidemic that screening has prevented in the UK', *The Lancet*, 2004, 364(9430): 249–256.

27. Janet E. Lane-Claypon, *Cancer of the Uterus: A Statistical Inquiry Into the Results of Treatment, Being an Analysis of the Existing Literature*, Reports on Public Health and Medical Subjects, no. 40, London: Ministry of Health, 1927, p. vi.

28. Angela E. Raffle, B. Alden, and E.D. Mackenzie, 'Detection rates for abnormal cervical screens: what are we screening for?', *The Lancet*, 1995, 345(8963): 1469–1473; Angela E. Raffle and M. Quinn, 'Harms and benefits of screening to prevent cervical cancer', *The Lancet*, 2004, 364(9444): 1483–1484.

29. Christopher Howson, Tomihiko Hiyama, and Ernst Wynder, 'The decline in gastric cancer: the epidemiology of an unplanned triumph', *Epidemiological Reviews*, 1986, 6: 1–27.

Chapter 6

1. Guilliame Vallée, *Dissertation sur le cancer de l'utérus*, Paris: Imprimerie Didot Jeune, 1826, p. 10.

2. Rigoni-Stern, 'Statistical facts relative to the disease of cancer', communication at sub-session on surgery of the Fourth Congress of Italian Scientists, 23 September 1842. Translated in: Joseph Scotto and John Bailard, 'Rigoni Stern and medical statistics: a nineteenth century approach to cancer research', *Journal of the History of Medicine and Allied Sciences*, 1969, 24(1): 65–75.

3. B. Ramazzini, 1713, *De Morbis Artificium (Diseases of Workers)*, Chicago: University of Chicago Press, 1940 (translation W.C. Wright).

4. Jacques Le Brun, 'Cancer serpit. Recherches sur la représentation du cancer dans les biographies spirituelles féminines du XVIIe siècle', *Sciences Sociales et Santé*, 1984, 2: 9–31.

5. J.C.W. Lever, 'Statistical notices on one hundred and twenty cases of carcinoma uteri', *Medico-Chirurgical Transactions*, 1839, 22: 267–273, on p. 270.

6. Louisa Garrett Anderson and Kate Platt, 'Malignant disease of the uterus. A digest of 265 cases treated in the New Hospital for Women', *Journal of Obstetrics and Gynaecology of the British Empire*, 1908, 14(6): 381–392, on p. 391.

7. E.F. Neve, 'Decade of tumor surgery in Kashmir', *Indian Medical Gazette*, May 1902, p. 164; C.R. Suryanarayan, 'Kangri cancer in kashmir valley: preliminary study', *Seminars in Surgical Oncology*, 2006, 5(4): 327–333.

8. The relationship between availability of medical care during childbirth and outcomes was complex. In the early twentieth century rich women treated by intervention-prone physicians often fared less well than middle-class ones, attended by the more conservative midwives, but still better than poor women who did not have access to any expert help. Irving Loudon, 'Maternal mortality: 1880–1950. Some regional and international comparisons', *Social History of Medicine*, 1988, 1(2): 183–228.

9. Frederick L. Hoffman, *Cancer in the North American Negro*, New York: P.B. Hoeber, 1931.

10. In hindsight it is probable that these families carried a genetic trait—a *BRCA* mutation—which made them especially susceptible to breast and ovarian cancers. Such mutations are frequent among Jews of East Europen origin.

11. Janet E. Lane-Claypon, *A Further Report on Cancer of the Breast. With Special Reference to Its Associated Antecedent Conditions*, London: Ministry of Health, 1926.

12. P. Weir and Clarence C. Little, 'The incidence of uterine cancer in Jews and Gentiles,' *Bulletin of the ASCC*, 1934, 16(2): 6–7.

13. W. Sampson Handley, 'The prevention of cancer', *The Lancet*, 1936, i: 987–991, on p. 990.

14. Georg Wolff, 'Cancer and race with specific reference to the Jews', *The American Journal of Hygiene*, 1939, 29(3): 121–137, on p. 136.

15. Xavier Castellsauge, Xavier Bosh, Nubian Munoz *et al.*, 'Male circumcision, penile human papilloma virus and cervical cancer in female partners', *New England Journal of Medicine*, 2002, 346(15): 1105–1112.

16. Joseph Menczer, 'The low incidence of cervical cancer in Jewish women: has the puzzle finally been solved?', *Israeli Medical Association Journal*, 2003, 5(2): 120–123.

17. C.E. Martin, 'Epidemiology of cancer of the cervix: II. Marital and coital factors in cervical cancer', *American Journal of Public Health*, 1967, 57: 803–814; I.D. Roitkin, 'Adolescent coitus and cervical cancer', *Cancer Research*, 1967, 27: 603–617.

18. J.W. Gardener and J.L. Lyon, 'Cancer of the cervix: a sexually transmitted infection?', *The Lancet*, 1974, ii: 470–471.

19. Brian E. Henderson, 'Sexual factors and pregnancy', in Joseph Fraumeni (ed.), *Persons at High Risk of Cancer: An Approach to Cancer Etiology and Control*, New York, Academic Press, 1975, pp. 267–283, on p. 279.

20. A. Singer, L.R. Bevan, and M. Coppelson, 'A hypothesis: the role of a high risk male in etiology of cervical carcinoma', *American*

Journal of Obstetrics and Gynecology, 1976, 34: 867–868; J.D. Buckley, R.W.C. Harris, R. Doll *et al.*, 'Case control study of the husbands of women with dysplasia or carcinoma of the cervix uteri', *The Lancet*, 1981, ii: 1010–1014.

21. I.D. Rotkin, 'A comparison review of key epidemiological studies in cervical cancer related to current research for transmissible agents', *Cancer Research*, 1973, 33: 1353–1367.

22. Harald zur Hausen, 'Human genital cancer: synergism between two virus infections or synergism between a virus infection and initiating events?', *The Lancet*, 1982, ii(8312): 1370–1372.

23. Harald zur Hausen, 'Condolomata acuminata and human genital cancer', *Cancer Research*, 1976, 36(2): 530; Harald zur Hausen, 'Human papillomaviruses and their possible role in squamous cell carcinomas', *Current Topics in Microbiology and Immunology*, 1977, 78: 1–30.

24. M. Durst, L. Gissmann, H. Ikenberg, and H. zur Hausen, 'A papillomavirus DNA from a cervical carcinoma and its prevalence in cancer biopsy samples from different geographic regions', *Proceedings of the National Academy of Science USA*, 1983, 80: 3812–3815; Richard Peto and Harald zur Hausen (eds), *Viral Etiology of Cervical Neoplasia*, New York: Cold Spring Harbour Laboratory Press, 1986.

25. Henderson, 'Sexual factors and pregnancy', p. 275.

26. Denise Leite Maia Monteiro, Alexandre José Baptista Trajano, Kátia Silveira da Silva, and Fábio Bastos Denise Russomano, 'Pre-invasive cervical disease and uterine cervical cancer in Brazilian adolescents: prevalence and related factors', *Cadernos de Saúde Pública*, 2006, 22(12): 2539–2548.

27. Rebecca Skloot, 'A nation obsessed with Jade Goody's cervical cancer but not mentioning why she's dying from it', 28 February 2009. http://scienceblogs.com/culturedish/2009/02/a_nation_obsessed_with_jade_go.php.

28. Jerome Groopman, 'Contagion: papilloma virus', *New Yorker*, 13 September 1999.

29. Spinelli's story can be found at http://thephoenix.com/boston/life/89069-living-with-hpv/.

30. See http://www.youtube.com/watch?v=tAmcFGORIcw for 2006 publicity and www.youtube.com/watch?v=Yj7aSivwgvM, for 2008 one.

31. See www.youtube.com/watch?v=f66nM-UbQQc.

32. European Cervical Cancer Association, *HPV Vaccination in Europe*, 2009. www.ecca.info/.../HPV_Vaccination/ECCA_HPV_Vaccination_April_2009.pdf.

33. H.L. Vu, S. Sikora, S. Fu, and J. Kao, 'HPV-induced oropharyngeal cancer, immune response and response to therapy', *Cancer Letters*, 2010, 288(2): 149–155; W.M. Mendenhall and H.L. Logan, 'Human papillomavirus and head and neck cancer', *American Journal of Clinical Oncology*, 2009, 32(5): 535–539.

34. Charlotte Haug, 'Human papilloma viruses: reasons for caution', *New England Journal of Medicine*, 2008, 359(8): 861–862, on p. 861.

35. Elisabeth Rosenthal, 'Drug makers' push leads to cancer vaccines' fast rise', *New York Times*, 20 August 2008.

36. Robert Aronowitz, 'Gardasil, a drug against individual risk', in Keith Wailoo, Julie Livingston, Steve Epstein, and Robert Aronowitz (eds), *Three Shots at Prevention: The HPV Vaccine and the Politics of Medicine's Simple Solutions*, Baltimore, MD: Johns Hopkins Univeristy Press, 2010, pp. 21–38, on p. 32.

Chapter 7

1. Nawal Naur, 'Cervical cancer: preventable death', *Reviews in Obstetrics and Gynecology*, 2009, 2(4): 240–249.

2. John Ehrenberg, 'Patient safety: first, do no harm', *PAHO Bulletin*, November 2004.

3. Lynette Denny, Louise Kuhn, Amy Pollack, and Thomas Wright, 'Direct visual inspection for cervical cancer screening', *Cancer*, 2002, 94(6): 1699–1707.

4. Rengaswamy Sankaranarayanan, Atul Madhukar Budukh, and Rajamanickam Rajkumar, 'Effective screening programmes for cervical cancer in low- and middle-income developing countries', *Bulletin of the World Health Organization*, 2001, 79(10): 954–962.

5. 'New method for cervical cancer prevention', *PAHO Bulletin*, December 2007.

6. Rengaswamy Sankaranarayanan, Bhagwan Nene, Surendra Shastri *et al.*, 'HPV screening for cervical cancer in rural India', *New England Journal of Medicine*, 2009, 360(14): 1384–1394.

7. Sankaranarayanan, Budukh, and Rajkumar, 'Effective screening programmes for cervical cancer', p. 960.

8. Jessica Gregg, 'Mixed blessing: cervical cancer screening in Recife, Brazil', *Medical Anthropology*, 2000, 19: 41–63, on pp. 46–47.

9. Luiz Claudio Santos Thuler, 'Mortalidade por câncer do colo do útero no Brasil', *Revista Brasileira do Ginecologia e Obstetrica*, 2008, 30(5): 216–218; Carmen Justina Gamarra, Joaquim Gonçalves Valente, and Gulnar Azevedo e Silva, 'Correction for reported cervical cancer mortality data in Brazil, 1996–2005', *Revista de Saude Publica*, 2010, 44(4): 629–638.

10. Clarissa Moraes de Sousa Bottari, Miguel Murat Vasconcellos, and Maria Helena Magalhães de Mendonça, 'Câncer cérvico-uterino como condição marcadora: uma proposta de avaliação da atenção básica', *Cadernos do Saúde Pública*, 2008, 24(supp. 1): S111–S122.

11. Nancy Scheper-Hughes, *Death Without Weeping: The Violence of Everyday Life in Brazil*, Berkeley, CA: California University Press, 1992.

12. Jessica Gregg, *Virtually Virgins: Sexual Strategies and Cervical Cancer in Recife, Brazil*, Stanford, CA: Stanford University Press, 2003.

13. Gregg, *Virtually Virgins*, p. 120.

14. Gregg, *Virtually Virgins*, p. 137.

15. Wilbur Sawyer, 'Medicine as a social instrument: tropical medicine', *New England Journal of Medicine*, 1951, 244(6): 217–224.

Epilogue

1. Julia Lawton, 'Contemporary hospice care: the sequestration of the unbound body and "dirty dying"', *Sociology of Health and Illness*, 1998, 20(2): 121–143.

2. www.naxos.com/education/opera_libretti.asp?pn=&char=AL L&composer=Berg&opera=Woyzeck&libretto_file=Libretto. htm [in German]. Berg's text is based on Georg Buchner's play *Woyzeck*, written in 1837; the lines about cancer were, however, added by Berg.

3. Jessica Gregg, *Virtually Virgins: Sexual Strategies and Cervical Cancer in Recife, Brazil*, Stanford, CA: Stanford University Press, 2003, p. 158.

4. Adonis de Carvalho, 'Câncer como problema de medicina tropical', *Revista Brasiliera de cancerologia*, 1967, 23(35): 65–89.

FURTHER READING

Prologue

Ada Lovelace has been the subject of serveral biographical studies: Doris Langley Moore, *Ada Lovelace, Byron's Legitimate Daughter*, New York: Harper and Row, 1977; Dorothy Stein, *Ada, A Life and a Legacy*, Cambridge, MA: The MIT Press, 1985; Joan Baum, *The Calculating Passion of Ada Byron*, Hamden, CT: Archon, 1986; Benjamin Wooley, *The Bride of Science: Romance Reason and Byron's Daughter*, New York: McGraw Hill, 1999. Dorothy Stein, in 'Lady Lovelace's notebooks: technical text and cultural context', *Victorian Studies*, 1984, 28(1): 33–67, attempted to investigate Ada Lovelace's contributions to mathematics, while her attitude to her own sick body was studied by Alison Winter in her article, 'A calculus of suffering: Ada Lovelace and the bodily constraints on women's knowledge in early Victorian England', in Christopher Lawrence and Steven Shapin (eds), *Science Incarnate: Historical Embodiments of Natural Knowledge*, Chicago: University of Chicago Press, 1998, pp. 202–239. Lovelace's letters, collected by Bette Toole in *Ada, The Enchanteress of Numbers: A Selection of Letters*, Mill Valley, CA: Strawberry Press, 1992, narrate the progress of her terminal disease.

Biographies of Eva Péron focus mainly on her political role. Her disease and death are discussed in George Sava, *Mourning Becomes Argentina*, Bognor Regis: New Horizon, 1978; John Barnes, *Evita First Lady: A Biography of Eva Péron*, New York: Grove

Press, 1978; Nicholas Faser and Marysa Navarro, *Eva Péron*, New York: WW Norton & Company, 1980; Alicia Dujovne Ortiz, *Eva Péron*, New York: St Martin Press, 1996. Jorge Albertelli's book, *Las 'Cien dias' de Eva Péron*, Buenos Aires: Cesarini Hermanos Editores, 1994, and Nelson Castro's book, *Los ultimos dias de Eva: Historia de un engano*, Buenos Aires: Vergara Editor, 2007, focus on Eva Péron's cancer, while Barron Lerner's 'The illness and death of Eva Péron: cancer, politics, and secrecy', *The Lancet*, 2000, 355: 1988–1991 investigates the politics of her treatment, seen from the USA.

Chapter 1

Female diseases in the Middle Ages were studied in Danielle Jacquart and Claude Thomasset, *Sexuality and Medicine in the Middle Ages* (translated by Matthew Adamson), Cambridge: Polity Press, 1988; Monica H. Green (editor and translator), *The Trotula: A Medieval Compendium of Women's Medicine*, Philadelphia: University of Pennsylvania Press, 2002; Monica Green, *Making Women's Medicine Masculine: The Rise of Male Authority in Pre-Modern Gynaecology*, Oxford: Oxford University Press, 2008; and Katharine Park, *Women's Secrets: Gender, Generation and the Origins of Human Dissection*, New York: Zone Books, 2006.

The origins of the present-day understanding of cancer are traced in Lelland J. Rather's book, *The Genesis of Cancer: A Study in the History of Ideas*, Baltimore, MD: Johns Hopkins University Press, 1978. See also Henry Sigerist, 'The historical development of pathology and therapy of cancer', *Bulletin of the New York Academy of Medicine*, 1939: 642–653; Alexander Haddow, 'Historical notes on cancer from the manuscripts of Louis Westenera Sambon', *Proceedings of the Royal Society of Medicine* (section on history of medicine), 1936, 29: 1015–1028. A useful, if not always fully reliable survey of early attitudes to cancer of the womb can be found in Michael O'Dowd and Elliot Philipps, *The History of Obstetrics and Gynacology*, New York: The Pantheon Group, 1944, pp. 543–570.

Nineteenth-century attitudes to incurable diseases are at the centre of Jason Szabo's book, *Incurable and Intolerable, Chronic Diseases and Slow Death in Nineteenth Century France*, New Brunswick, NJ: Rutgers University Press, 2009. Female diseases in the nineteenth century are investigated in Ann Douglas Wood, '"The fashionable diseases": women's complaints and their treatment in nineteenth century America', *Journal of Interdisciplinary History*, 1973, 4(1): 25–52 and Carroll S. Rosenberg and Charles E. Rosenberg, 'The female animal: medical and biological views of women in the nineteenth century', *Journal of American History*, 1973, 60: 332–356. Karen Nolte's article, 'Carcinoma uteri and sexual debauchery: morality, cancer and gender in the nineteenth century', *Social History of Medicine*, 2008, 21(1): 31–46, examines doctors' beliefs on links between gynaecological cancers and supposedly immoral sexual conduct.

Chapter 2

The history of gynaecology and gynaecological surgery in the nineteenth century were studied by Ornella Moscucci in her book, *The Science of Woman: Gynaecology and Gender in England, 1800–1929*, Cambridge: Cambridge University Press, 1990 and in George Weisz in his, *Divide and Conquer: A Comparative History of Medical Specialization*, New York: Oxford University Press, 2006. Moscucci also investigated the view of cancer as a female disease in Ornella Moscucci, 'Gender and cancer in Britain, 1860–1910',

American Journal of Public Health, 2005, 95(8): 1312–1321. Patrice Pinell investigated the passage from the understanding of cancer of the womb as an incurable condition to its redefinition as a curable ailment in Patrice Pinell, *The Fight Against Cancer*, London: Routledge, 2002.

Stephen Jacyna described relationships between surgeons and pathologists in the nineteenth century in Stephen Jacyna, 'The laboratory and the clinics: the impact of pathology on surgical diagnosis in Glasgow Western Infirmary, 1875–1910', *Bulletin of the History of Medicine*, 1988, 62: 384–406. On the history of biopsy and microscopic diagnosis of cancer see George Rosen, 'Beginnings of surgical biopsy', *American Journal of Surgical Pathology*, 1977, 1(4): 361–364; James Wright, 'The development of the frozen section technique, the evolution of surgical biopsy, and the origins of surgical pathology', *Bulletin of the History of Medicine*, 1985, 59: 295–326; Ilana Löwy, 'Breast cancer and the "materiality of risk": the rise of morphological prediction', *Bulletin of the History of Medicine*, 2007, 81: 241–266; Ilana Löwy, *Preventive Strikes: Women, Precancer and Preventive Surgery*, Baltimore, MD: Johns Hopkins University Press, 2010, chapter 1.

Regina Morantz-Sanchez's book, *Conduct Unbecoming a Woman: Medicine on Trial in Turn-of-the-Century Brooklyn*, Oxford: Oxford University Press, 1999, focuses on the career of the New York surgeon Mary Amanda Dixon Jones and provides at the same time a carefully researched and nuanced historical overview of the development of gynaecology and gynaecological surgery in late nineteenth-century USA. Details of Louisa Garrett Anderson's surgical career can be found in Jennian F. Geddes' 'Louisa Garrett Anderson (1973–1943): surgeon and suffragette', *Journal of Medical Biography*, 2008, 16: 205–214.

Chapter 3

The history of radium in France was studied by Soraya Boudia in her book, *Marie Curie et son laboratoire: sciences et industrie de la radioactivité en France*, Paris: Éditions des Archives Contemporaines, Paris, 2001. Works on the history of radiotherapy and radiation therapy include Manuel Lederman, 'The early history of radiotherapy, 1895–1939', *International Journal of Radiation Oncology, Biology and Physics*, 1981, 7: 639–648; Bénédicte Vincent, 'Genesis of the Pavillon Pasteur of the institut Du Radium of Paris', *History and Technology*, 1997, 13(4): 293–305; Charles R.R. Hayter, 'The clinic as laboratory: the case of radiation therapy, 1896–1920', *Bulletin of the History of Medicine*, 1998, 72(4): 663–688; Ton van Helvoort, 'Scalpel or rays? The struggle for cancer patients in pre-war II Germany', *Medical History*, 2001, 45: 33–60; John Pickstone, 'Contested cumulations: configurations of cancer treatment through the twentieth century', *Bulletin of the History of Medicine*, 2007, 81: 164–196.

Janet Lane-Claypon's pioneering statistical work is described in Warren Winkelstein, 'Vignettes of the history of epidemiology: three firsts by Janet Elisabeth Lane-Claypon', *American Journal of Epidemiology*, 2004, 160(2): 97–101; Ellen Leopold and Warren Winkelstein, 'Unsung heroines: unveiling history, Janet Elisabeth Lane-Claypon', *Breast Cancer Action Newsletter*, no. 81, May–June 2004; Nigel Paneth, Ezra Susser, and Mervyn Susser, 'Origins and early development of case control study. Part 2, The case control study from Lane-Claypon to 1950', *Sozial und Preventivemedizin*, 2002, 47: 359–365. Ornella Moscucci's article, '"The ineffable masonery of sex": feminist surgeons and the establishement of radiotherapy in early twentieth century Britain', *Bulletin of the History of Medicine*, 2007, 81: 139–163, provides a detailed study of early uses of radiotherapy for treatment of gynaecological cancers in the UK.

Chapter 4

The history of the Pap smear was investigated by Monica J. Casper and Adele E. Clarke, 'Making Pap smear into the "right tool" for the job: cervical cancer screening in the USA, circa 1940–1995', *Social Studies of Science*, 1998, 28(2): 255–290; Adele E. Clarke and Monica J. Casper, 'From simple technology to complex arena: classification of Pap smears, 1917–1990', *Medical Anthropology Quarterly*, 1996, 10(4): 601–623; and by Eftychia Vayena, *Cancer Detectors: An International History of the Pap Test and Cervical Cancer Screening, 1928–1970*, unpublished PhD thesis, University of Minnesota, 1999.

Lynda Bryder's book, *Women's Bodies and Medical Science: An Inquiry Into Cervical Cancer*, Basingstoke: Palgrave Macmillan, 2010, is a detailed (but for some controversial) analysis of the controversy on the treatment of cervical cancer in the Women's National Hospital in New Zealand. Pamela Hyde's paper, 'Science frictions: cervical cancer and the contesting of medical beliefs', *Sociology of Health and Illness*, 2000, 22(2): 217–234, provides an additional analysis of this controversy. Yolanda Ergaso examined the history of colposcopy in Latin America in 'Migrating techniques, multiplying diagnoses: the contribution of Argentina and Brazil to cervical cancer "early detection" policy', *Manguinhos*, 2010, 17(suppl. 1): 33–51.

Sociological and anthropological reflections on the meaning of screening for women include Vicky Singleton and Mike Michael, 'Actor networks and ambivalence: general practitioners in the UK Cervical Screening Programme', *Social*

Studies of Science, 1993, 23(2): 227–264; Linda McKie, 'The art of surveillance or reasonable prevention? The case of cervical cancer screening', *Sociology of Health and Illness*, 1995, 17: 441–457; Patricia A. Kaufman, 'Screening the body: the Pap smear and the mammogram', in *Living and Working with the New Medical Technologies*, Margaret Lock, Allan Young, and Alberto Cambrosio (eds), Cambridge: Cambridge University Press, 2000, pp. 165–183; Anette Forss, Carol Tishermann, Catarina Widmark, and Lisbeth Sachs, 'Women's experiences of cervical cellular changes: an unintentional transition from health to liminality?', *Sociology of Health and Illness*, 2004, 26(3): 306–325.

Chapter 5

In her book *Early Detection: Women, Cancer, and Awareness Campaigns in the Twentieth-Century United States*, Chapel Hill, NC: University of North Carolina Press, 2006, pp. 53–92, Kirsten Elizabeth Gardner examines US interwar campaigns to promote an early detection of cervical cancer. Post-Second World War US campaigns are described in Eftychia Vayena *Cancer Detectors: An International History of the Pap Test and Cervical Cancer Screening, 1928–1970*, unpublished PhD thesis, University of Minnesota, 1999. UK campaigns were discussed by Elisabeth Toon in a talk entitled 'Demand and supply, success and failure: managing the provision of cervical cancer screening in the 1960s UK' to the conference How Cancer Changed, Paris, 2–4 April 2009, and studied by Ilana Löwy in *Preventive Strikes: Women, Precancer and Preventive Surgery*, Baltimore, MD: Johns Hopkins University Press, 2010, chapter 5. Ornella Moscucci analysed cancer education in the UK in her paper 'The British fight against cancer: publicity and education, 1900–1948', *Social History of Medicine*, 2010, 23(2): 356–373.

Problematic aspects of the early detection of cancer are discussed by Gilbert Welch, *Should I Be Tested For Cancer? Maybe Not, and Here's Why*, Berkeley, CA: University of California Press, 2004, while Louise B. Russell's book, *Is Prevention Worse Than Cure?*, Washington DC: The Brookings Institution, 1986, explains why screening campaigns which have a sound scientific basis can still be inefficient. Lynda Bryder's article, 'Debates about cervical screening: an overview', *Journal of Epidemiology and Community Health*, 2008, 62: 284–287, summarizes recent controversies on the efficacy of screening for cervical tumours.

Chapter 6

Joseph Scotto and John Bailar III, 'Rigoni Stern and medical statistics: a nineteenth century approach to cancer research', *Journal of the History of Medicine*, 1969, 24(1): 65–75, and Malcolm Griffiths, '"Nuns, virgins and spinsters": Rigoni Stern and cervical cancer revisited', *British Journal of Obstetrics and Gynaecology*, 1991, 98: 797–802, look at Rigoni-Stern's early studies. Keith Waloo discusses the links between race and cervical cancer in *How Cancer Crossed the Colour Line*, NY: Oxford University Press, 2011, chapter 2.

The collective volume, *Three Shots at Prevention: The HPV Vaccine and the Politics of Medicine's Simple Solutions*, edited by Keith Wailoo, Julie Livingston, Steve Epstein, and Robert Aronowitz (Baltimore, MD: Johns Hopkins University Press, 2010), provides a broad perspective on recent controversies surrounding the introduction of the HPV vaccine. Additional elements on this topic can be found in James Colgrove's 'The ethics and politics of compulsory HPV vaccination', *New England Journal of Medicine*, 2006, 33(23): 2389–2391; Monica Casper and Laura Carpenter, 'Sex, drugs and politics: HPV vaccine for cervical cancer', *Sociology of Health and Illness*, 2008, 30(6): 886–899; and Laura Carpenter and Monica Casper, 'Global intimacies: innovating the HPV vaccine for women's health', *Women's Studies Quaterly*, 2009, 37(1–2): 80–100.

The Wellcome Witness Seminar, *History of Cervical Cancer and Papilloma Virus, 1960–2000*, edited by Lois Reynolds and E.M. Tansey (Wellcome Trust Centre at UCL, 2008), is a rich source of information on the development of HPV studies in the UK.

Chapter 7

The relative invisibility of cervical cancer in developing countries is attested to by the paucity of secondary literature on this topic. A notable exception is Jessica Gregg's important book, *Virtually Virgins: Sexual Strategies and Cervical Cancer in Recife, Brazil*, Stanford, CA: Stanford University Press, 2003, discussed in this chapter.

The history of cancer control in Brazil is described by Luiz Antonio Teixeira and Cristina M. Fonseca, *De Doença Desconhecida a problema de saúde pública: o Inca e o controle do câncer no Brasil*, Rio de Janeiro: Ministério da Saúde, 2007. Nancy Scheper-Hughes's book, *Death Without Weeping: The Violence of Everyday Life in Brazil*, Berkeley, CA: California University Press, 1992, is focused on maternal and child health in poor zones of the Brazilian north east.

INDEX